The Arthritis Foundation's

Guide to Good Living With Rheumatoid Arthritis

SECOND EDITION

ARTHRITIS
FOUNDATION®
Take Control. We Can Help.™

Published by
Arthritis Foundation
1330 West Peachtree Street
Suite 100
Atlanta, GA 30309
www.arthritis.org

Printed in Canada
1st Printing 2004

Library of Congress Card Catalog Number: 2004107995

ISBN: 0-912423-46-3

Acknowledgments

The Arthritis Foundation's Guide to Good Living with Rheumatoid Arthritis, Second Edition is written for people who have rheumatoid arthritis, as well as for their friends, family and loved ones. Bringing this book to completion was a team effort, including the significant contributions of dedicated physicians, health care professionals, Arthritis Foundation volunteers, writers, editors, designers and Arthritis Foundation staff.

Special acknowledgments should go to the medical editor of the original edition of this book, Theodore Pincus, MD, Professor of Medicine at Vanderbilt University School of Medicine, as well as to his co-editor, Cynthia M. Kahn. The chief medical reviewer of the book is John H. Klippel, MD, Chief Executive Officer of the Arthritis Foundation.

The panel of reviewers of this book are rheumatologists Joan Bathon, MD, Johns Hopkins Bayview Medical Center, Division of Rheumatology, Baltimore, MD; Marcy Bolster, MD, Medical University of South Carolina, Division of Rheumatology and Immunology, Charleston, SC; Doyt L. Conn, MD, Emory University School of Medicine and Grady Health System, Division of Rheumatology/Immunology, Atlanta, Ga.; and Mary Corr, MD, University of California, San Diego, School of Medicine. In addition, Jennifer Lewis, an Arthritis Foundation volunteer who also has rheumatoid arthritis, reviewed the original edition of this book for accuracy from the patient's perspective. Additional thanks go to Gretchen Henkel, who served as a writer on the early stages of the book's development.

Editorial directors of this book are Susan Bernstein and Elizabeth Axtell. The cover design is by Matthew Lennert. The interior design is by Jill Dible, who also served as the production artist. The art director of the book is Tracie Bullis.

Table of Contents

It is difficult, impossible really, to make comparisons among the 100 or more different forms of arthritis. Each touches the lives of persons affected in very personal and often profound ways.

However, by whatever standard one might choose, rheumatoid arthritis ranks high on the list of the most serious forms of arthritis. Although it can begin at any age – including childhood – young women in the prime of their lives are most commonly affected. Joint pain and limitations become a daily experience, and interfere with essentially all activities – both those needed to simply make it through the day as well as pleasurable activities. Moreover, for most people, the arthritis becomes chronic and persists for their entire lifetime. Over the course of years, rheumatoid arthritis leads to damage to joints and deformities of hands, wrists and other joints, further limiting a person's ability to use their joints.

For many people with rheumatoid arthritis, the uncertainty of knowing what the future holds and the frustration that drugs or other approaches to treatment have provided little relief of symptoms, pose major challenges. Fortunately, this situation is changing rapidly, particularly over the past decade, which has witnessed remarkable progress in the scientific understanding of rheumatoid arthritis. Research is beginning to provide important clues that have already resulted in newer, more highly effective drugs to treat the disease. Ongoing and future research will teach us a great deal about the disease, yet to be able to truly cure or even prevent rheumatoid arthritis seems a real and distinct possibility.

The Arthritis Foundation believes that the actions people with rheumatoid arthritis choose to take play a large and important role in determining the outcome of the disease, and the extent to which it impacts their lives. Education, self-help and taking personal responsibility are tools of empowerment - all keys to working effectively with physicians to achieve control of rheumatoid arthritis. This book, *The Arthritis Foundation's Guide to Good Living with Rheumatoid Arthritis, Second Edition* is a resource guide for people with rheumatoid arthritis, as well as their families and loved ones, to help in the understanding of this disease, and improve their lives.

John H. Klippel, M.D.
Chief Executive Officer
Arthritis Foundation, Atlanta, GA

Part One

Rheumatoid Arthritis:
Understanding the Disease

Chapter 1

Understanding
Arthritis:
Clearing Up Myths and Exploring Treatment Approaches

The goal of this book is to give you strategies and information that can help you achieve good living with rheumatoid arthritis. Before we get started, though, it's necessary to take a step back and look at the big picture. This chapter may be used as a building block for understanding the complex condition known as rheumatoid arthritis, sometimes abbreviated as RA.

"Arthritis" is a term derived from the Greek words "arth" (meaning joint) and "itis" (meaning inflammation). The literal meaning of the word is "joint inflammation." However, the word arthritis is often used to refer to any of the more than 100 different conditions that cause pain in the joints and tissues surrounding them, such as muscles and tendons (which connect muscles to bone). These conditions may be called forms of arthritis, musculoskeletal conditions or rheumatic diseases. In many sources – including this book – these terms are used interchangeably.

The physicians who specialize in diagnosing and treating arthritis and related rheumatic diseases are called *rheumatologists*. People who experience symptoms such as joint pain or swelling may not initially seek the care of a rheumatologist, because they may not know that they should. They may make an appointment with their regular, primary-care physician, such as an internist or family physician. Or, they may schedule an appointment with an *orthopaedist*, a doctor who specializes in treating bone disorders and ailments. These physicians can refer patients to a rheumatologist if necessary for diagnosis or treatment. Children can also have forms of arthritis, including juvenile rheumatoid arthritis. These children should seek diagnosis and treatment from a pediatric rheumatologist if at all possible. These physicians specialize in the treatment of juvenile rheumatic diseases in children and adolescents.

Arthritis Myths

Arthritis has been recognized for perhaps thousands of years. Even prehistoric skeletal remains of humans show signs of arthritis. Unfortunately, the myths about arthritis have been around for almost as long. We will try to debunk some of these myths about arthritis and provide some key definitions along the way.

Major Arthritis Myths

Arthritis is just another name for joint aches and pains associated with aging.

Arthritis isn't really a serious health problem.

Not much can be done to help people with arthritis.

MYTH #1: ARTHRITIS IS JUST ACHES AND PAINS

One common myth is that arthritis is just another name for the aches and pains everyone gets as we get older. While it is true that arthritis becomes more common as people age, arthritis may begin at any age, including childhood. Some elderly people never develop arthritis. Many forms of arthritis or musculoskeletal conditions are self-limited and get better without specific treatment. Others, such as rheumatoid arthritis, may be quite serious and may affect the body's internal organs as well as the joints.

A simple way to organize arthritis-related conditions is to group them into categories based on whether they affect only one joint or area of the body (localized conditions) or many joints and organs over the entire body (generalized conditions), as shown in the box. Localized conditions include two sub-groups. The first subgroup includes conditions that affect the soft tissues surrounding joints and bones, but do not affect the structure of joints or bones directly. These are known as soft-tissue, localized conditions, and include *tendinitis* and *bursitis*. The second subgroup includes conditions that affect one or a few joints, such as a single knee or hip. A common example of this second subgroup is osteoarthritis of a single joint, although osteoarthritis often affects more than one joint.

Likewise, generalized conditions can be divided into two subgroups. In the first subgroup, widespread muscle and soft tissue discomfort in which there is no evidence of swelling or inflammation includes a very common condition called *fibromyalgia*. Conditions in this subgroup are not associated with damage to the structure of the joints. The second subgroup includes condi-

Arthritis-Related Conditions

Localized conditions
(affect one joint or one area of the body)

- Soft tissue localized conditions (bursitis or tendinitis, for example)
- Conditions that affect one or a few joints (such as osteoarthritis)

Generalized conditions
(affect many joints or areas of the body)

- Widespread muscle/soft tissue conditions without inflammation (such as fibromyalgia)
- Inflammatory conditions usually involving joints (rheumatoid arthritis, psoriatic arthritis, gout, vasculitis and ankylosing spondylitis)

tions in which inflammation affects the entire body, such as rheumatoid arthritis. Other conditions in this subgroup include gout, ankylosing spondylitis and psoriatic arthritis, generalized conditions of inflammation throughout the body in which joint pain is the major symptom. Other generalized inflammatory conditions include polymyositis, which affects primarily muscles; systemic lupus erythematosus (lupus), which may affect the skin, kidney or other organs; and vasculitis, which may affect any organ.

These four groups of musculoskeletal conditions are not mutually exclusive, and a person may have more than one type of rheumatic disease. For example, people with rheumatoid arthritis may experience tendinitis, bursitis and fibromyalgia more commonly than people in the general population. In addition, when joints become badly damaged as a result of the chronic inflammation of

rheumatoid arthritis, they are called "end stage." At this point, they may look similar to joints that have reached "end stage" in people with osteoarthritis, even though the destruction was caused by different mechanisms.

MYTH #2: ARTHRITIS ISN'T REALLY A SERIOUS HEALTH PROBLEM

Arthritis and related rheumatic diseases, as well as chronic joint symptoms, are the most common chronic health conditions in the population, affecting about 70 million Americans. These conditions become even more common among older people. Even in people under age 65, arthritis is a major cause of work disability. For example, fewer than 50 percent of rheumatoid arthritis patients younger than 65 who are working at the onset of the disease are still working ten years later.

In addition, the impact of arthritis on society is substantial. By recent estimates calculated by the Centers for Disease Control, the costs associated with arthritis may amount to $86 billion annually – putting the economic impact of arthritis on a par with a moderate recession! The costs of arthritis may be categorized into three groups: direct, indirect and intangible. *Direct* medical costs, such as physician (and other health professional) fees, charges for laboratory tests and X-rays, drugs, assistive devices, surgeries and other costs, are the most obvious. However, a substantial part of the economic burden are *indirect* costs, such as lost wages due to work disability. In addition, people experience *intangible* costs, such as the need for a spouse or relative to take time off from work to bring a patient to a caregiver, travel for medical care, or money spent to remodel the home to meet the needs of a person with arthritis, and many others.

MYTH #3: NOT MUCH CAN BE DONE TO ALLEVIATE THE PAIN AND DISABILITY OF ARTHRITIS

Unfortunately, there are no "cures" for most chronic rheumatic conditions. You may think that little can be done to help your arthritis. This simply is not true: Some improvement in the pain and loss of function is possible in almost everyone with arthritis. Furthermore, the disease process that may lead to joint destruction can be controlled effectively in most people – particularly those with rheumatoid arthritis. More can be done today to ease the pain of arthritis and to slow joint destruction than ever before. The first step to take is to see a qualified doctor and get an accurate diagnosis.

Many people with serious types of arthritis, which were severely disabling as recently as a generation ago, are now leading full and productive lives thanks in part to many developments including new drugs and treatments, exercise programs, surgeries and self-management. Your future, as a person with arthritis, is full of possibilities that were only a dream 25 years ago.

One of the most exciting changes in recent years has been the growing understanding that the patient has an important role to play in the management of his or her arthritis. This change in emphasis is sometimes referred to as a *biopsychosocial model* of disease management, to distinguish it from the traditional *biomedical model*, in which the outcomes of diseases are thought to be determined almost exclusively by the actions of health professionals. Of course, the wonderful advances in drugs, surgeries and other medical treatments are an important component of a biopsychosocial model of disease management, but this model also incorporates the key contribution of patients, families and support networks to the outcome. In the second part of this chapter, we will focus on this model, which lays the groundwork for many of the ideas expressed throughout the remainder of this book.

The Biopsychosocial Model for Arthritis Care

The biomedical model of medical care evolved in the late 19th and early 20th century and was based on the idea of identifying a single cause and cure for each disease. This model was extremely successful and is still used. It works well when doctors care for people with acute infections, such as pneumonia; acute surgical conditions, such as appendicitis; and conditions affecting a single organ, such as a heart attack. Many of our ideas and expectations of medical care are based on the success of this approach, which relies heavily on high technology tests and state-of-the-art treatments that lead to cures.

As chronic diseases and health problems have come to the forefront at the beginning of the 21st century, certain limitations of the biomedical model have become clear. First, the causes and treatments of chronic diseases are complex – there is rarely one cause or one "cure." Second, people who have chronic diseases have important contributions to make to the outcomes of their disease – the results appear to be influenced as much by the actions of the patient as by the actions of the doctor or other health professionals. In fact, there is growing evidence that much of the key information for making a diagnosis, predicting the outcome and monitoring chronic disease comes directly from the patient in the form of patient histories and questionnaires. These are, of course, supplemented by the knowledge of health professionals and information gained through high technology tests.

In recognition of the importance of the patient's role, new management strategies have evolved to supplement the traditional biomedical approach. Collectively, these strategies have come to be known as a biopsychosocial model, which includes the idea that chronic conditions involve an intermingling of many factors – including biological, psychological and socioeconomic – that can affect the course and outcome of disease.

This approach emphasizes that people who have chronic diseases should become knowledgeable about the consequences of disease and effects of therapy, and should understand the importance of *self-management* in disease outcomes. Self-management refers to actions by the patient that may favorably affect the course and outcome of chronic disease. By combining active self-management strategies with the information and treatment available from doctors and other health professionals, people with arthritis may experience greater benefits – such as increased pain relief and a better quality of life – than those who do not become involved in their own care. Some specific principles of the biopsychosocial approach are summarized in the box on p. 5

Principles of Arthritis Management

1. Each person is an individual and should be viewed as a "person with a type of arthritis," rather than as a "type of arthritis seen in a person."

2. There is no "best treatment" for everyone who has a particular type of arthritis, as each individual may respond differently to different treatments.

3. No single type of arthritis is always "better" or "worse" than another type.

4. Information and input from a person with arthritis can be as valuable in diagnosis and management as information from laboratory tests and X-rays.

5. In arthritis management, the emphasis is on improving function of joints and relieving pain.

6. Your doctor and health-care team need your involvement to help you to the fullest extent – people with arthritis and health professionals are partners in care.

7. Something can always be done your situation with arthritis.

and are discussed here. These principles create the foundation on which this book is based, and they will be referred to frequently in the following chapters.

1. EACH PERSON IS AN INDIVIDUAL AND MUST BE VIEWED AS A "PERSON WITH A TYPE OF ARTHRITIS," RATHER THAN AS A "TYPE OF ARTHRITIS IN A PERSON."

When a doctor deals with an acute problem, such as a specific type of pneumonia, there is usually a standard course of treatment that varies little from person to person. While each patient's case is unique, in acute events, the biomedical model usually works well. However, in a chronic disease such as rheumatoid arthritis, doctors use a more individualized approach. Each person may need a different combination of medications, exercise, therapy and devices to achieve the best quality of life.

2. THERE IS NO "BEST TREATMENT" FOR EVERYONE WHO HAS A PARTICULAR TYPE OF ARTHRITIS, AS EACH INDIVIDUAL MAY RESPOND DIFFERENTLY TO DIFFERENT TREATMENTS.

In a chronic disease such as arthritis, there can be no "best" treatment for all people, because each person experiences his or her own individual set of symptoms and disease course. In addition, different people may experience very different responses to some of the drugs frequently used to treat arthritis. One person may find a particular medication to be extremely useful, while a sec-

ond person may get no benefit at all from the same drug. A third might even have adverse effects from the drug and not be able to continue taking it. We hope you will always ask your health professional about new treatments and whether they might work for you. However, it's important to understand that there is no single "best" treatment for everyone.

3. NO SINGLE TYPE OF ARTHRITIS IS ALWAYS "BETTER" OR "WORSE" THAN ANOTHER TYPE.

Sometimes people ask, "Is rheumatoid arthritis worse than osteoarthritis?" or the other way around. It's true that, on average, some types of arthritis may cause more pain or disability than other types. However, arthritis affects each individual differently, and no type of arthritis is invariably better or worse than another type. For example, someone who has bursitis of the hip may experience more discomfort and functional disability than someone with a mild form of rheumatoid arthritis or osteoarthritis.

Some factors that contribute to the severity of the disease include:

• How the condition affects your daily life, including the ability to take care of yourself or continue to work;
• How you react to symptoms of pain, fatigue, disability and psychological distress; and
• How you respond to treatments, including possible side effects.

Any or all of these can affect how you and the health professionals managing your care perceive the severity of your arthritis.

4. INFORMATION FROM A PERSON WITH ARTHRITIS CAN BE AS VALUABLE IN DIAGNOSIS AND MANAGEMENT AS INFORMATION FROM LABORATORY TESTS AND X-RAYS.

In the traditional medical approach, doctors rely heavily on tests and data to diagnose and monitor a condition. These tests are often quite valuable in chronic diseases such as rheumatoid arthritis, but most important information is obtained directly from the patient. In fact, there is no single "test" that can diagnose or confirm most types of arthritis. When talking to your doctor, *you* can provide the most important clues by answering the questions that are part of your patient history. In caring for chronically ill or debilitated people, doctors need to listen

Personally Speaking Stories from real people with rheumatoid arthritis

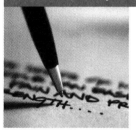

"I just got back from the doctor's office where I have been pre-diagnosed with rheumatoid arthritis. I had to go to the hospital for some more blood tests to be positive about the diagnosis, and then I go to a specialist. My first reaction was one of sadness. I couldn't help but cry. My grandfather has lived most of his adult life with this disease, but I was always told it was a reaction to bullet shrapnel from the war.

Diagnosis: My First Reactions
by Melissa Anderson, Portage, Michigan

"I think about the pain my Grandpa has gone through and I can't bear it. I would do almost anything to be able to take this away from him. Now that I am in the process of being diagnosed with arthritis, I have no choice but to take this head on. I am scared of my life ahead. I am afraid I won't be able to lift and carry the children I someday want to have. I am afraid I won't be able to cut my own food. I am afraid of watching my body become deformed. I am afraid I won't be able to afford to take care of myself. My Grandpa is 88, and I am hoping and praying that I have just a little bit of his strength and will power so that I can live through this pain.

"The first person I told was my mom. She said, 'Everything will be OK.' I think this is what I needed to hear. She also told me not to tell anyone at work, that it could be a problem down the road with promotions and insurance. That wasn't exactly what I wanted to hear.

"Tonight, I will sit down with my boyfriend and look up more information about this disease on the Internet. We are moving into our first apartment together this Saturday, and I am afraid this disease will make me different from who I am now."

to more than just physical symptoms or test results. Your doctor may also use a short questionnaire or diagram to get more information about your arthritis and how it affects your daily life and activities.

5. IN ARTHRITIS MANAGEMENT, EMPHASIZE IMPROVING FUNCTION OF JOINTS AND RELIEVING PAIN.

The strategy in many illnesses is to try to get test measures, such as blood pressure, blood sugar (glucose) or cholesterol levels back into the normal range. In rheumatoid arthritis, your strategy should be to improve function, relieve pain, find coping strategies and deal with everyday physical and emotional problems related to the disease. Although the goals do include getting blood tests, such as an elevated erythrocyte sedimentation rate (ESR or sed rate) or C-reactive protein (CRP) into the normal range (see Chapter 4), your emphasis should be on how you function from day to day. Your daily well-being should tell you more about the progress of your treatment than your X-ray or lab test result.

6. YOUR DOCTOR AND HEALTH-CARE TEAM NEED YOUR INVOLVEMENT IN ORDER TO HELP YOU TO THE FULLEST EXTENT – PEOPLE WITH ARTHRITIS AND HEALTH PROFESSIONALS ARE PARTNERS IN CARE.

If someone is acutely ill, the doctor may be expected to provide almost all the "management," such as determining which tests

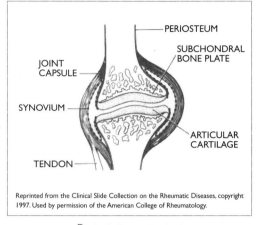

Reprinted from the Clinical Slide Collection on the Rheumatic Diseases, copyright 1997. Used by permission of the American College of Rheumatology.

DIAGRAM OF A HEALTHY JOINT

are needed, selecting a treatment and administering these treatments. In a hospital, the doctor writes "orders" and treatments are provided by the hospital staff. The patient has no responsibility for treatment, other than taking the medicine and cooperating with the prescribed therapy.

In a chronic disease, your doctor and other health-care professionals can "manage" only a small component of your care. You need your doctor to diagnose your illness and prescribe treatment, but you're in control 99 percent of the time – spending less than a few hours each month or even each year with doctors and other health-care professionals. To get the best results, you must be a very active participant in your own care. This approach is called *self-management*, and it's the cornerstone of this book.

The first thing to do if you experience symptoms is to see a doctor and get a proper diagnosis. But once you have that diagnosis, you and your doctor, and other health-care professionals you consult, must act as a team. You – not your doctor – are ultimately in control of whether and when to take a medication, do exercises, practice good joint protection techniques or take any other steps toward controlling arthritis. Your actions and attitude will determine the success of your treatment.

7. SOMETHING CAN ALWAYS BE DONE TO IMPROVE LIFE WITH ARTHRITIS.

You've heard some of the attitudes about life with arthritis: "Arthritis is inevitable," or "Oh, it's arthritis – there's nothing you can do about it except learn to live with the pain."

These attitudes are out of date. There is *always* something that can be done to improve a situation for a person with arthritis. It may be a new drug, a new surgical technique, a device to make tasks easier, an exercise, a support group or maybe even a book like this one.

Don't expect a miracle. Instead, focus on hard work and determination to make your life with arthritis more productive and enjoyable. Most treatments require some trade-off: time and effort spent on exercise, the cost of a new drug or device, or medication side effects. However, you can be optimistic that your situation can be improved, because it always can!

Chapter 2

Rheumatoid Arthritis:

The Basics of a Chronic, Complex Disease

Rheumatoid arthritis (*def.*): A chronic disease in which inflammation of the joints (and sometimes other parts of the body) leads to long-term damage, which may result in chronic pain, loss of function and disability.

I‌f you have rheumatoid arthritis, you've probably heard something similar to the definition above from your doctor. Perhaps you have wondered what all these terms mean. In this chapter, we're going to break down this definition into easily understood sections, and we hope to give you a better understanding of what happens in this complicated condition. We'll also give you some information about the history of rheumatoid arthritis, ongoing research into its possible causes and what it's like to have this disease.

Understanding Rheumatoid Arthritis

RHEUMATOID ARTHRITIS IS CHRONIC

Rheumatoid arthritis is a chronic disease because once you develop it, it will continue relatively indefinitely and not go away. It can begin either suddenly or gradually. In some people with rheumatoid arthritis, particularly early in the disease, all signs of their arthritis gradually disappear. This is called a *spontaneous remission*. However, if a spontaneous remission occurs, it is usually seen within six months of the onset of symptoms and swelling. If the pain and swelling continue for longer than six months, you're likely to develop a persistent or chronic condition.

Occasionally, people with rheumatoid arthritis may experience attacks of joint swelling that occur every few weeks or months, but then totally subside after only a few days. There may be no evidence of any arthritis between these attacks. This is known as *palindromic rheumatism*. (A palindrome is a phrase that reads the same forward and backward, such as "Madam I'm Adam.") About one half of people who experience palindromic rheumatism go on to develop chronic rheumatoid arthritis, with its characteristic persistent inflammation. Others continue to experience self-limited attacks for many years. In a lucky few, these attacks may even disappear.

Chronic diseases are best diagnosed and monitored using a patient-centered approach. In this approach, input from the person with arthritis is considered at least as, if not more, important as laboratory tests. Treatment is complex, usually involving a combination of drugs and other measures over time, rather than a single drug. And the person with the illness is a critical part of the disease-management team, using self-help measures, including mind-body approaches, to manage the disease day to day.

In fact, health-care professionals are generally "in control" of a person's chronic disease less than one-tenth of one percent of the time, or less than one hour per month. Most of the time, managing your chronic disease is your responsibility. Learn as much as you can about your particular disease, its potential course and available treatments. Be proactive in monitoring your symptoms and treatments and in handling the day-to-day challenges your disease brings. Rely on your doctor for treatment prescriptions and advice, but manage your own health and care.

RHEUMATOID ARTHRITIS INVOLVES INFLAMMATION

When the body is threatened by some type of foreign "invader," such as an infec-tion, it normally mounts a response known as *inflammation* to help fight this threat. The chemicals released by the body to fight the infection cause a reaction that stimulates fever, swelling and associated pain – typical signs of inflammation.

In rheumatoid arthritis, inflammation of joints causes them to become swollen, tender and painful. But in rheumatoid arthritis, inflammation occurs throughout the body, so organs such as the eyes or lungs may be affected as well. People with rheumatoid arthritis often experience fatigue and flu-like symptoms.

For the most part, the early joint inflammation that occurs in rheumatoid arthritis is reversible. However, if unrecognized and untreated, uncontrolled inflammation – seen as chronic swelling and tenderness of joints – may lead to irreversible joint damage. Such damage can be documented on X-rays. Although each person experiences a different disease course, damage may begin in many people as early as the first year of disease. Joint damage caused by inadequately controlled inflammation can lead to loss of joint movement, decreased ability to work, higher medical costs and potential surgery. That's why it's so important to get a diagnosis as soon as possible and to begin a course of drug treatment to control inflammation. Newly developed treatments, such as biologic response modifiers, can control inflammation and prevent joint damage if given early enough in the course of the disease (see Chapter 11).

RHEUMATOID ARTHRITIS INVOLVES AN ABNORMAL IMMUNE SYSTEM RESPONSE

Several types of white blood cells are involved in the immune system response. One type of specialized white blood cell is known as a B-lymphocyte: a cell that produces *antibodies* directed to neutralize foreign substances known as *antigens*. These antibodies and antigens combine into what are known as "immune complexes," which are then removed by scavenger cells. Another class of cells are called T-lymphocytes, which regulate the function of B-cells by suppressing or stimulating the production of antibodies.

The immune system normally protects the body from disease through an elaborate network of signals that control the production of antibodies when needed, and turn off this production when they are no longer needed. Normally, this elaborate control system works very well to maintain your health. But in rheumatoid arthritis, the signals don't function properly. The immune system mistakenly views the body as the foreign invader, a process known as *autoimmunity*. The immune cells then attack the body, causing inflammation that results in later damage to joints and other organs.

One interesting example of the incorrect signal referred to above is known as *rheumatoid factor*. Rheumatoid factor is an antibody that is directed to regulate normal antibodies made by an individual. Rheumatoid factor is a type of "anti-antibody," which may

be normal in small quantities when the signals of the immune system function properly. However, excess amounts of rheumatoid factor may be seen when the signals do not function properly.

Although most people with rheumatoid arthritis do have rheumatoid factor, it may not be found early in the disease. And some people with severe rheumatoid arthritis never have rheumatoid factor. However, rheumatoid factor is one very important discovery in establishing that the immune system is incorrectly programmed in rheumatoid arthritis, leading to recent advances in treatments.

The immune system has been – and continues to be – the subject of much research. Many potential therapies for rheumatoid arthritis and other autoimmune diseases aim to "correct" the faulty signals that distort the immune response, and/or to overcome their consequences.

Who Gets Rheumatoid Arthritis?

It is estimated that rheumatoid arthritis affects about 0.5 percent to 1 percent of the population in the United States and most countries around the world. That's about 2.1 million Americans. Rheumatoid arthritis may begin at any age. RA affects infants and the elderly, as well as those in the prime of life. However, more than 70 percent of people with rheumatoid arthritis are women, and the most common onset is between the ages of 40 and 50.

What Causes Rheumatoid Arthritis?

Despite extensive research for decades, the cause of rheumatoid arthritis remains unknown. Scientists have learned much about the immune response and the mechanisms of inflammation in arthritis (see the beginning of this chapter), but the actual triggering events that start the abnormal process remain a mystery.

Historically, RA was considered to be "chronic infectious arthritis," because its disease features were similar to those seen in infectious diseases like tuberculosis. However, extensive efforts to identify a specific infectious agent (such as a bacterium, fungus or virus) that may cause rheumatoid arthritis have failed to pinpoint a culprit. More recently, researchers have tried to identify the "footprints" of an agent (such as the genetic material or DNA of an infectious agent) in the tissue of people with rheumatoid arthritis. To date, these studies remain inconclusive.

Even if a single infectious agent or footprints of such an agent were found consistently in people with rheumatoid arthritis, it is unlikely that everyone infected with this agent would get rheumatoid arthritis. The genetic makeup of an individual influences whether or not that individual develops an infection with any agent, even the common flu virus. Therefore, even if an infectious agent is found in most people with rheumatoid arthritis, the basis of why that person develops the disease would be explained only in part, with a need to look at other factors that contribute to the disease.

It is possible that what is now called rheumatoid arthritis actually includes many different diseases that are grouped together under the same name at this time. This has happened many times in the history of medicine. For instance, 150 years ago physicians recognized only one or a few types of pneumonia. Today, dozens of types of pneumonia have been described and categorized. Similarly, as more is learned about rheumatoid arthritis, many different diseases may be recognized as falling under its general umbrella.

THE ROLE OF GENDER

One important clue to the origin of rheumatoid arthritis is gender. As noted earlier, more than 70 percent of people with rheumatoid arthritis are women. This observation has led to theories that gender may play some part in what causes rheumatoid arthritis and its severity.

Many women with rheumatoid arthritis experience improvement in their symptoms during pregnancy. Furthermore, rheumatoid arthritis develops more often than expected in the year after a pregnancy, and after a baby is born, women may experience an increase in symptoms. However, the understanding of possible effects of female hormones in rheumatoid arthritis remains limited at this time.

THE ROLE OF OTHER GENETIC FACTORS

In addition to gender, considerable progress has been made over the last 20 years in identifying specific genes that may be linked to an increased risk of developing rheumatoid arthritis. One such factor is known as the major histocompatibility antigen, which is found on the surface of lymphocytes and is known as HLA, human lymphocyte antigen. The HLA genetic site, or *locus*, controls immune responses. Researchers have shown that people with a specific genetic marker – known as the HLA shared epitope – have a fivefold greater probability of developing rheumatoid arthritis than people without the marker. More than two-thirds of Caucasian people with rheumatoid arthritis have this genetic marker, compared to only about 20 percent of the general population.

Although this genetic marker is associated with increased risk of disease and may be an important clue in the cause of rheumatoid arthritis, it cannot be used as a diagnostic test. This is because only a small minority of people with the shared epitope actually develop rheumatoid arthritis. In addition, many people with rheumatoid arthritis do not have this genetic marker.

Further research suggests that other, yet-to-be-identified genes influence the development of disease as well. Researchers continue to search for these genes by identifying

Personally Speaking Stories from real people with rheumatoid arthritis

After Diagnosis: I Keep Moving
by Carlene Fiorito,
East Providence, RI

"I was diagnosed in October 2003 with rheumatoid arthritis. I suffered for three years beginning the day after the birth of my son. After years of wrong diagnoses, I was finally diagnosed with rheumatoid arthritis after limping around in horrible pain for more than six months.

"I've tried several treatments over the last six months and I'm currently on *Remicade*. I am a 36-year-old female who has always been very active and in good health. To help ease my pain, I take yoga classes and exercise regularly using my treadmill and other light floor exercises.

"My husband and family have been very supportive. They often help me with housework and keep my spirits up with their concern and care. If it weren't for my twin sister helping me in every way, I'm not sure where I would be. I also read a lot and I'm proactive in my disease treatment. I am constantly doing research on my own on helpful tips to live and cope with RA. I eat a healthy diet, drink no caffeine, and even when I feel like I can't get out of bed because of severe fatigue, I keep moving!!

"My faith in God and something much bigger than me gets me through each and every day."

families in which several members may have arthritis and analyzing their DNA (which makes up the genetic code).

NEW INSIGHTS

There have recently been new insights to suggest that stress may play a role in rheumatoid arthritis. A *stress* in this case can refer to a physical trauma, emotional upheaval or anything that stimulates the body to produce a stress response. Some researchers have suggested that rheumatoid arthritis may begin or worsen at times of stress.

Normally, the central nervous system responds to stress by sending out a complicated series of signals resulting in the production of *corticosteroids* by the body's adrenal glands. So a stressful stimulus should lead to an increase in corticosteroid levels. However, some people with rheumatoid arthritis appear to have a "blunted" response to stress, causing them to produce lower levels of corticosteroids. This may explain why people with rheumatoid arthritis often respond dramatically to small doses of corticosteroid drugs such as prednisone.

What Is it Like To Have Rheumatoid Arthritis?

All this information about the process of inflammation and what happens inside your body at a cellular level doesn't tell you what RA feels like on a daily basis. Let's discuss the common symptoms you may experience with this disease.

First of all, remember that the specific problems of one person with rheumatoid arthritis may differ greatly from those of another person. The most common symptoms of RA include:

- Stiffness (especially in the morning)
- Fatigue
- Pain
- Swelling in multiple joints

While any joint may become involved, people commonly first experience symptoms of joint inflammation in the knuckles of the hands, the feet and the wrists. In some people with RA, the elbows, shoulders, hips and knees become involved as well.

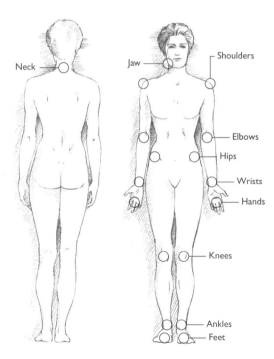

JOINTS THAT MAY BE AFFECTED BY RHEUMATOID ARTHRITIS

A summary of the joints most likely affected by rheumatoid arthritis can be found in the diagram on page 16. In addition, the box on this page provides some key definitions that will help you understand the structure of your joints and how they are affected by inflammation.

In addition to physical symptoms, people with RA often experience psychological stress, frustration, helplessness and loss of control as they learn to cope with the day-to-day effects of this chronic disease. Psychological problems can, in turn, make it more difficult to cope with their arthritis. Pain may even get worse. The good news is that you can do something about the cycle of pain and depression. Getting proper treatments and developing new skills – on your own or with the help of others – to cope with pain and stress in positive, constructive ways can help you fight that spiraling cycle.

Although arthritis is a chronic disease, you can control your symptoms. The good news is that the severe consequences seen in people with rheumatoid arthritis may now be prevented in most people. People with rheumatoid arthritis can feel more optimistic about their future than ever before. Drugs that are more effective and have fewer side effects than traditional medications are available now. These drugs are often used earlier in the disease, and in combination with one another, bringing about more effective control of inflammation. Exercise programs, joint protection activities and a

number of self-management techniques can significantly help people take control of their rheumatoid arthritis. All of these strategies will be discussed later in this book.

So, be informed, be proactive, but above all, be optimistic. You *can* achieve good living with rheumatoid arthritis.

Your Joints: A Marvel of Engineering

A *joint* connects one bone to another. Joints come in various shapes and sizes: some move like a hinge (your finger and knee joints, for example); others have a "ball in socket" structure that allows them to move in many directions (your shoulder and hip joints); still others move in several different directions (your wrist and ankle). There are more than 70 moveable joints in the human body – and rheumatoid arthritis can affect any of them.

Other soft-tissue structures surround the joint and may also be affected by arthritis. *Ligaments* are flexible bands of fibrous tissue that connect bones to one another. *Muscles* consist of fibers that stretch and tighten, allowing movement of the body's organs and joints. At the ends of muscles are the *tendons* that connect muscle to bone.

If you looked inside a joint, you would find *cartilage*, a smooth substance that lines the joint so your bones do not wear each other down. The *synovial fluid* found in the joint (the *synovium* is the lining of the joint) lubricates it and allows free movement. When joints are actively inflamed, inflammatory cells are found in the synovial fluid and synovial lining, and cause breakdown of cartilage and bone.

Chapter 3

Diagnosing
Rheumatoid Arthritis:
Your Medical History and Physical Examination

D iagnosis is the first step on the road to proper treatment and control of rheumatoid arthritis. RA symptoms often occur suddenly, causing confusion for the person affected. As no single laboratory test instantly confirms an RA diagnosis, doctors must use a variety of methods to determine the cause of patients' symptoms. Let's shed some light on the processes that doctors use to diagnose rheumatoid arthritis. The more you know about these methods – and the importance of the information you can provide – the better you will become at understanding and participating in the process.

RA differs from other diseases such as diabetes or kidney disease, in which very specific and simple blood tests can confirm the diagnoses in most people. By contrast, the rheumatoid factor (the antibody discussed in the previous chapter whose presence may indicate rheumatoid arthritis) test is positive in many people with rheumatoid arthritis, but is negative in 20 percent to 30 percent of the people who have this disease. Furthermore, a test for rheumatoid factor may be positive in people who do not have rheumatoid arthritis.

Even discovering which kind of arthritis a person has is not always easy. As we discussed in Chapter 1, each person experiences his or her own individual disease course, and a person may have more than one type of rheumatic condition at the same time. A skilled physician will use the information provided by the patient and the findings of a physical examination to decide a likely diagnosis, and then determine which tests are needed. In fact, the most important parts of the diagnostic process are a careful medical history, including a full discussion of current symptoms, and a complete physical exam. Tests do not always provide a clear answer.

The "Low-Tech" Tools

It should be no surprise to you that the practice of medicine has become very "high tech" in recent years. Batteries of tests and the use of expensive imaging equipment have become standard. However, in rheumatoid arthritis, the most important and perhaps surprising tools for diagnosis are the "low-tech" components of your office visit – your medical history and physical examination.

MEDICAL HISTORY

Ever wonder why you have to fill out forms and answer so many questions when you visit your doctor? No, it's not just a plot to distract you while you wait for the nurse to call you in – you're actually providing important clues to help your doctor make a proper diagnosis. Some of the key questions that you may be asked during your initial office visit include:

• **Do you have joint pain in many joints?** People who have rheumatoid arthritis usually experience joint involvement in several joints at once, as opposed to having pain in only one joint.

• **Does the pain occur symmetrically – that is, do the same joints on both sides of your body hurt at the same time? Or is the pain one-sided?** Symmetric pain is often a sign of rheumatoid arthritis. For instance, if both wrists are swollen, or the same knuckles in both hands, rheumatoid arthritis may be likely.

• **Do you have stiffness in the morning?** Morning stiffness, another hallmark of rheumatoid arthritis, occurs when the joints feel stiff and are difficult to move. Doctors are often interested in how long your morning stiffness lasts. After a period of loosening up, motion becomes easier and less painful. Stiffness is likely to recur after sitting for prolonged periods of time.

• **When is the pain most severe?** For example, do your joints hurt more in the morning or late in the day? Inflammation, like that seen in rheumatoid arthritis, often is associated with joints feeling better with moderate activity, but greater discomfort may occur in the early morning and later in the day, when fatigue sets in.

• **Do you have pain in your hands, wrists and/or feet?** Although rheumatoid arthritis can occur in any joint of the body, these joints are most frequently involved and cause symptoms of pain and swelling.

• **If you have pain in your hands – if so, which joints hurt the most?** In rheumatoid arthritis, rows of joints such as those where your fingers make their first bend (metacarpophalangeal joints) and the middle knuckles of the fingers (proximal interphalangeal joints) tend to be affected more often than the knuckles near the tips of the fingers.

• **Have you had periods of feeling weak and uncomfortable all over? Do you feel fatigued?** Many people with rheumatoid arthritis notice generalized problems, such as muscle aches, fatigue, stiffness, weight loss and a general "flu-like" feeling.

Your answers to these and other questions often let the doctor know if rheumatoid arthritis should be considered as a diagnosis. And, if you have already been diagnosed with rheumatoid arthritis, your medical history will continue to play a starring role in your office visits, as your doctor will want to keep close tabs on your pain and functional status, any developing limitations in your abilities to perform activities, your medications, and any side effects you may experience.

PATIENT QUESTIONNAIRES

Patient self-report questionnaires, in addition to the medical history, are increasingly used by doctors to provide critical information about your disease course and treatment. Some of the most important problems experienced by people with rheumatoid arthritis, including loss of function, pain, fatigue and psychological distress, are not measured directly by any blood test, X-ray or other high-tech measure. Therefore, doctors use the results from patient question-

Personally Speaking Stories from real people with rheumatoid arthritis

"I had only been married about six months when all of my symptoms started. I started with extreme pain in my wrists and ankles. I was very fatigued all of the time. I had absolutely no energy. I'm a first grade teacher and my job requires constant attention to my students. I had to stay on my feet constantly and I knew I was having a hard time even having enough energy to make it through the day.

Starting Over: A First Grade Teacher's Tale
by Sherry Collier, Wylliesburg, VA

"I went to several different doctors trying to find out what my problem was. My doctor wanted to say that it was depression. I knew my body better than anyone else, and I knew it was more than just depression. Yes, I was depressed because no one could tell me what my physical problem was.

"After many tests, I was referred to a rheumatologist who did more tests and finally concluded that one of my major problems was that I had RA. My doctor started me on medicine that has helped me so that I can work every day. Sometimes the days are pretty long but I do my best to hang in there.

"Not only do I have RA, but I have also been diagnosed with multiple sclerosis. Needless to say, each day is a true challenge. I am very fortunate that I have a wonderful family that has been there for me throughout this long ordeal. I give thanks also to my doctor who never gave up on finding the cause of my problems. Most of all, I thank God for each new day with its challenges and the strength to see me through."

naires to assess the impact of rheumatoid arthritis on daily life.

If your doctor is not currently using a patient questionnaire, you may want to consider discussing it with him or her, because these measures have been proven to be one of the most effective ways to monitor changes in disease over a five- to 10-year period. Several self-report questionnaires have been tested and widely used in the care of people with rheumatoid arthritis. Two of the most common are described below.

• **The Health Assessment Questionnaire (HAQ).** This measurement tool includes 20 activities of daily living in eight categories including dressing, eating, walking and other activities. Participants are also asked to measure their pain and their overall outlook, and to answer questions about their use of aids and devices. Modified versions (modified HAQ, and multidimensional HAQ) have been developed to provide additional data within a two-page format that includes global status, measures of fatigue and psychological distress, and medication review.
• **The Arthritis Impact Measurement Scales (AIMS).** This tool includes several dimensions of health status including mobility, physical activity, dexterity, household activities, anxiety, depression and social activities, in addition to activities of daily living and pain.

PHYSICAL EXAMINATION

After your medical history, a thorough physical examination by a doctor knowledge-able about rheumatoid arthritis will usually supply most of the necessary information to make a diagnosis. Your doctor will look for common features of RA, including:

• **Joint swelling.** This may be severe or barely noticeable. A skilled doctor should be able to recognize even slight joint swelling that may indicate rheumatoid arthritis.
• **Joint tenderness.** Certain joints may be painful to even the slightest touch.
• **Loss of motion in your joints.** This may indicate inflammation (see Chapter 2 for a description of the inflammatory process) or joint damage. The physician will assess your joints' range of motion; for instance, can you move your shoulders through a complete circle?
• **Joint malalignment.** After several years of rheumatoid arthritis (especially if inflammation is unchecked), some joint damage often occurs, causing joints to be out of alignment. This is most commonly seen in the small joints of the hands and feet.
• **Signs of rheumatoid arthritis in other organs.** Rheumatoid arthritis is a *systemic* disease, meaning it may affect other systems in your body. The doctor will look for involvement in other parts of the body including your skin, lungs and eyes, among others.

The doctor will review each joint during the physical exam to determine which joints have signs of arthritis, including tenderness, pain on motion, swelling, limited motion and long-term damage. *Joint counts* have been shown to be quite useful to assess, monitor and predict the course of rheumatoid arthritis in individuals. Usually, your doctor will not only make a complete count of which joints are involved, but also will assess the severity of the involvement in each joint.

PHYSICAL MEASURES OF FUNCTION

Your doctor may want to get an idea of your ability to perform certain tasks. Physical function measures may indicate both evidence of inflammation and evidence of long-term damage. A member of your doctor's office staff, or a physical or occupational therapist may perform these tests. Some widely used measures include the following:

• **Grip strength.** The traditional method for measuring grip strength has been to inflate a blood pressure cuff (30 mmHg) and ask the individual to squeeze as hard as possible, first with the right then with the left hand. The pressure change on the cuff is recorded. The test is usually repeated several times.

• **Walking time.** The individual is asked to walk a set distance (usually 25 or 50 feet) at a normal pace. The time to complete the distance is then recorded.

• **Button test.** The individual is asked to unbutton and button five buttons as quickly as possible using a standard button board. The score is recorded in seconds.

CLASSIFICATION CRITERIA

You may have heard or read about something called "classification criteria for

---

Classification Criteria for Rheumatoid Arthritis

These very specific classification criteria were developed by members of the American College of Rheumatology. The criteria describe patterns of symptoms that are *most commonly* seen in people with rheumatoid arthritis. They can be used as guidelines, but they will not give you or your doctor specific information about your prognosis (what will happen over time with your condition).

Classification Criteria
1. Morning stiffness
2. Arthritis of three or more joints
3. Arthritis of more than two hand joints
4. Symmetrical arthritis
5. Subcutaneous (rheumatoid) nodules
6. Rheumatoid factor
7. Radiographic (X-ray) changes

Adapted from Revised Classification Criteria for Rheumatoid Arthritis, *Arthritis and Rheumatism*, 1988, Volume 31, pp. 315-324, by Arnett, Edworthy, Bloch, et al.

---

rheumatoid arthritis" (see box). They were developed by a committee of rheumatologists (doctors who specialize in treating arthritis) and provide a guideline to the patterns of findings usually seen in rheumatoid arthritis.

Summary

As you can see, your doctor is able to obtain most of the valuable information needed to make a diagnosis of rheumatoid arthritis before a laboratory test is ever ordered. Your contribution can be substantial by providing clear and accurate information on your own medical history, as well as any family history of arthritis or joint symptoms. Keep track of which joints have been swollen or painful, because the disease may abate in some joints and flare in others over time.

Lab tests can provide additional important information to your doctor to make a diagnosis. We'll discuss these tests in the next chapter.

Chapter 4

Diagnosing
Rheumatoid Arthritis:

Laboratory Tests and Imaging Studies

Like the pieces of a puzzle, the information and clues that you and your doctor uncover will fit together in a way that will help determine whether or not you have rheumatoid arthritis. As you may already know from previous chapters, there is currently no laboratory test that can absolutely determine whether or not you have rheumatoid arthritis.

People with rheumatoid arthritis can have normal test results, and people can have abnormal test results yet not have rheumatoid arthritis. Interpretation of laboratory tests depends on the symptoms of the individual. So answering your doctor's questions honestly is key.

Some of the tests discussed in this chapter may be familiar to you. Others are used less commonly and may not be necessary for you. At times you may feel that you are looking into a bowl of alphabet soup as you ponder the importance of your ESR, RF, ANA and MRI, among others. But all of these tests can provide important clues when used in the right way.

When These Tests Are Helpful

Laboratory tests and imaging procedures can help your doctor confirm your diagnosis. In addition, they may help determine the severity of disease activity. Be aware that your doctor may choose to order only one or two tests discussed in this chapter, or he or she may use a test not described here. In general, you will not need to have most tests again after the diagnosis is made. Other tests, designed to check for drug side effects or to measure improvement, may need to be repeated at regular intervals.

Laboratory Tests Used in Diagnosis

COMPLETE BLOOD COUNT

Doctors measure levels, or counts, of different types of blood cells to assess patients with many types of diseases. There are three cellular components of blood: red blood cells carry oxygen to tissues, white blood cells help the body fight infections, and platelets help stop bleeding and form clots. Doctors often measure these cells during the first office visit. They may repeat this test during treatment to monitor for possible side effects from drugs and, sometimes, to check progress in reversing abnormalities.

Doctors measure red blood cells according to measures of hemoglobin, hematocrit and a red blood cell count. *Hemoglobin* is the protein in red blood cells that carries oxygen from the lungs to the tissues; it may be low in rheumatoid arthritis because of the "anemia of chronic disease." Similarly, the *hematocrit* (which measures the volume of red blood cells) and the red blood cell count (which measures the number of red blood cells) may be lower than normal in people with rheumatoid arthritis. The anemia seen in people with rheumatoid arthritis may contribute to feelings of fatigue or malaise. People with more aggressive disease tend to have more severe anemia.

Your doctor may also count your levels of white blood cells. A high white cell count may mean that an infection is present and can be a sign of severe inflammation. However, the white blood cell count is usually normal in people with rheumatoid arthritis, unless a simultaneous infection is present. (The white cell count may be low in an unusual complication of rheumatoid arthritis called Felty's syndrome, which we'll discuss later.) Some of the medications used to treat rheumatoid arthritis may cause a reduction in the white cell count, thereby reducing the body's capac-

ity to fight infections. So doctors will often monitor white blood cell count periodically in people with rheumatoid arthritis.

Platelets are small cells that participate in the formation of blood clots. Severe inflammation may elevate the platelet count, or certain drugs may depress it. The platelet count, along with the white blood cell count, are monitored about every six months in people who take only nonsteroidal anti-inflammatory drugs (NSAIDs), such as ibuprofen and naproxen, and about every two to 12 weeks in people who take most disease-modifying antirheumatic drugs (DMARDs), such as methotrexate and leflunomide.

ERYTHROCYTE SEDIMENTATION RATE

The erythrocyte sedimentation rate, also known as ESR or *sed rate*, is a valuable test often used to assess the degree of inflammation. The test is a measurement of how fast red blood cells (erythrocytes) fall to the bottom of a glass tube that is filled with blood and allowed to sit for one hour. People with any type of inflammation, including rheumatoid arthritis, often have higher sed rates than those in the normal range. If the level of inflammation is reduced with treatment, the sed rate usually drops. Because it is so important to control inflammation in rheumatoid arthritis, doctors may repeat this test fairly frequently.

One problem is that the ESR is elevated in only about 60 percent of people who have rheumatoid arthritis – meaning that the remaining 40 percent have a normal sedimentation rate. Remember: Your treatment is generally directed by the severity of your clinical symptoms, such as pain and functional ability. Therefore, even if your ESR is normal, treatment for your rheumatoid arthritis often should continue.

C-REACTIVE PROTEIN

C-reactive protein (or CRP) is another substance found in the body that indicates the presence of inflammation. Elevated levels of this protein provide an additional measure of disease activity in rheumatoid arthritis. Although the ESR and CRP often reflect similar degrees of inflammation, sometimes ESR levels are elevated when CRP levels are normal (and vice versa). This phenomenon is not well understood.

Some researchers have recognized that CRP levels that remain high over a long period are often associated with more severe joint damage later in the disease. This provides a strong rationale for trying to reduce the CRP to normal levels. However, some people with normal levels of CRP may still experience progressive joint damage.

As with the sedimentation rate, treatment for rheumatoid arthritis usually should continue even if CRP levels are normal. Your doctor may repeat this test at regular intervals to monitor the level of inflammation and your response to medication.

RHEUMATOID FACTOR

Some abnormal *antibodies* (special proteins produced by B-lymphocytes of the immune system in response to substances such as infectious agents) are found in the blood of people with rheumatoid arthritis that are not commonly found in people without the disease.

Rheumatoid factor (RF) is an antibody found in the blood of about 70 percent to 80 percent of people with rheumatoid arthritis. It is found in the serum component of the blood – the other half of the blood from the cellular components discussed above as red blood cells, white blood cells and platelets. It is an antibody directed to normal antibodies, as discussed in Chapter 2. These antibodies are normally produced by the body and are known as gamma globulins or immunoglobulin G (IgG).

Most people with rheumatoid arthritis have a large amount of rheumatoid factor circulating in the blood. However, the rheumatoid factor test is not a specific diagnostic test for rheumatoid arthritis. At least one in five people with rheumatoid arthritis does not have rheumatoid factor, but does have a form of the disease that cannot be distinguished from people who have rheumatoid factor.

People with rheumatoid arthritis who do not have rheumatoid factor in their blood or serum are often referred to as "seronegative." As noted, their disease doesn't differ from that of "seropositive" people who have rheumatoid factor in their serum. The rheumatoid factor test, also called the rheumatoid arthritis latex test, measures the amount of these antibodies in *titers* or units.

A titer is simply a number to indicate the dilution of blood at which rheumatoid factor may be detected, so that if the titer is 1:160, there is twice as much rheumatoid factor as if the titer is 1:80. Rheumatoid factor may also be measured in units – higher numbers mean more rheumatoid factor. However, test results may be negative during the first several months, making this test less useful in early diagnosis of rheumatoid arthritis. Nonetheless, this test for rheumatoid factor is eventually positive in 60 percent to 80 percent of people with rheumatoid arthritis.

Experts once thought that people with RA who had a positive rheumatoid factor test were more likely to have a severe disease course. Recent studies suggest that the differences in disease severity between those who do and do not have rheumatoid factor are not necessarily as great as researchers once believed.

ANTINUCLEAR ANTIBODIES

Another test for abnormal antibodies is called the antinuclear antibody (ANA) test. It detects a group of *autoantibodies* (antibodies against self) that combine with the nuclei of cells. These particular antibodies are most often positive in people with systemic lupus erythematosus (also known as SLE or lupus), but they are also seen in about 30 percent to 40 percent of people with rheumatoid arthritis. In addition, a positive ANA test may be seen in people with scleroderma (systemic sclerosis),

polymyositis and other inflammatory rheumatic diseases.

It is important to be aware that most people with positive antinuclear antibody tests have neither rheumatoid arthritis nor lupus, and probably have no disease at all. Because of the difficulty of interpreting meaningful results, many doctors no longer routinely use this test in diagnosing rheumatoid arthritis.

GENETIC TYPING

In recent years, much attention has been focused on the search for genetic markers that may predispose certain people to develop (or be susceptible to) a particular disease. About two-thirds of people with rheumatoid arthritis have a genetic marker known as a *shared epitope* at the major histocompatibility locus (see Chapter 2), or the area where the genes that control the immune system response are located.

Although identification of this shared epitope is critical for research studies to understand how rheumatoid arthritis develops, we must recognize that about seven percent of the normal population have the shared epitope but do not develop rheumatoid arthritis. At least 20 percent of people with rheumatoid arthritis do not have the shared epitope. So measurement of the epitope is not useful in diagnosing rheumatoid arthritis, since it will often give incorrect impressions.

URINALYSIS

A routine study done on the urine (urinalysis or UA) includes tests for sugar (which can identify and monitor diabetes), protein (seen when kidney abnormalities are present) or abnormal cells that indicate inflammation or infection of the kidney, bladder or other parts of the urinary tract. A urinalysis is not helpful in the diagnosis of rheumatoid arthritis, but it is used regularly in people with rheumatoid arthritis who are treated with certain medications such as gold or penicillamine. These drugs may cause damage to the kidneys in a few patients, so monitoring is necessary.

Imaging Studies

RADIOGRAPHS (X-RAYS)

X-rays taken early in the course of rheumatoid arthritis can show swelling of the soft tissues and loss of bone density around the joints because of both the patient's reduced activity and inflammation. In later disease, about 70 percent of people with rheumatoid arthritis will develop *erosions* (small holes) near the ends of bones and narrowing of the joint space due to loss of cartilage.

Personally Speaking   Stories from real people with rheumatoid arthritis

Aggressive Approach: Simple Coping, Strong Support
by Linda Shull, Charlotte, NC

"When symptoms first appeared as foot pain followed by wrist pain, I strongly suspected I might have RA. I was no stranger to RA. My mother has RA, as did my grandfather and great-grandfather. So, I had inside information about the disease.

"I started aggressive treatments very soon after my diagnosis was confirmed by a rheumatologist. Needless to say, my activities and abilities were affected. I had to teach my high school history classes in bedroom slippers and have students carry my book bag from my car to my classroom. Activities like aerobics and skiing were replaced with walking my dog and swimming. I was able to continue teaching full time for four more years.

"My strategies for coping with RA are simple. Though I wouldn't have chosen to have RA, it is the hand I have been dealt. My family and friends have been essential for my success in living well with RA. When I told my husband (one month after our wedding) that I would need a hip replacement, he became the solid rock of support I knew he would be. His steadfastness in 'sickness and health' was tested far earlier than he had expected, but his love and compassion have never wavered.

"Also, close friends circled the wagons and tirelessly volunteered comfort, cheer and understanding. They signed up for the harder labor – cooking, cleaning and taxi service – whenever I needed them. Overall, I have chosen to live as normally as my health permits. I have made RA a part of my life, not the focus of my life. I am blessed that I have many people in my life who help me do that every day."

Doctors once believed that they should delay aggressive drug treatment of RA until erosions were visible, because of the potential side effects. Visible erosions would absolutely confirm a rheumatoid arthritis diagnosis. Today, doctors use the opposite approach, treating RA aggressively and early before there is damage to joints caused by erosions. So X-rays are not necessarily used as guides to initiate treatment, but they remain important in evaluating how well certain treatments may control joint damage, and to help recognize when people may be candidates for joint surgery.

X-rays taken early in the disease course can provide a valuable baseline for comparison with later X-rays to see if and how the disease may progress. Many authorities have proposed that people with rheumatoid arthritis should have routine X-rays of the hands and feet every one to two years.

BONE SCANS

Bone scans may be used to detect evidence of inflammation in the body, including joints. While bone scans may be used to confirm the presence of *polyarthritis* (arthritis affecting multiple joints), this condition can usually be detected in a physical examination. Therefore, bone scans are generally not necessary to make a diagnosis of rheumatoid arthritis.

MAGNETIC RESONANCE IMAGING (MRI)

An MRI scan can detect early inflammation before X-ray changes are seen. These scans are effective at pinpointing *synovitis* (inflammation of the lining of the joint) in many people who show no damage on X-rays. MRI scanning is becoming an important diagnostic aid and method for monitoring the degree of arthritis activity in a joint or joints.

JOINT ULTRASOUND

Joint ultrasound is a much less expensive way to look for joint inflammation before X-rays show damage. Although not currently used often, this procedure may gain wider use over the next few years as doctors increase their efforts to document early evidence of disease.

BONE DENSITOMETRY

Bone densitometry is an important imaging study for measuring bone density, used primarily to detect *osteoporosis* – a major clinical problem for older people, particularly women. Osteoporosis may be especially severe in people with rheumatoid arthritis due to joint immobilization, the inflammatory response itself, and the use of certain therapies (corticosteroids) that may hasten bone loss. Some doctors suggest that a bone density test should be part of the evaluation and monitoring of all people with rheumatoid arthritis, particularly for women after menopause.

Chapter 5

Diagnosis
Checkpoints:

What if It's *Not* Rheumatoid Arthritis?

For the majority of people with rheumatoid arthritis, establishing a diagnosis can be done with confidence. But even skilled rheumatologists on occasion may have difficulty determining whether a person has rheumatoid arthritis or one of several other diseases that can have similar symptoms.

Diagnosis is not always a simple journey to a clear destination. When large groups of patients are studied over long periods of time, about five percent of people who were originally diagnosed as having rheumatoid arthritis actually turn out to have another type of rheumatic disease five to 10 years later. Another five percent of people who were thought to have other rheumatic diseases may turn out to have rheumatoid arthritis!

What is recognized today as rheumatoid arthritis probably involves many different types of diseases (see Chapter 2). In the future, physicians may well be able to distinguish several different forms of rheumatoid arthritis. This may partly explain why a diagnosis of rheumatoid arthritis can be associated with such variation in the number of joints or organs affected, the severity of symptoms, and the way the disease responds to therapy.

In this chapter, we take a look at some of the many other types of rheumatic diseases whose symptoms can sometimes mimic or resemble rheumatoid arthritis (see Diseases That Can Resemble Rheumatoid Arthritis, p. 32). Some of these diseases can even occur together with rheumatoid arthritis, making it even more important to obtain an accurate diagnosis, and determine appropriate treatment.

Osteoarthritis

Osteoarthritis (sometimes called *degenerative joint disease*) occurs when joint cartilage is worn away, causing damage and eventual destruction of the joint. This condition was once thought to be an inevitable part of getting old, and certainly the chance of developing it increases with age. However, many people never develop osteoarthritis, and many

Diseases That Can Resemble Rheumatoid Arthritis

Osteoarthritis *

Fibromyalgia*

Gout

Ankylosing spondylitis

Bursitis and Tendinitis*

Sjögren's syndrome*

Felty's syndrome *

Polymyalgia rheumatica

Connective Tissue Diseases:

   Systemic lupus erythematosus (lupus)

   Scleroderma

   Polymyositis/Dermatomyositis

   Vasculitis

* indicates disease/syndromes that may occur commonly together with rheumatoid arthritis.

Reprinted from the Clinical Slide Collection on the Rheumatic Diseases, copyright 1997. Used by permission of the American College of Rheumatology.

EROSIVE OSTEOARTHRITIS

people with osteoarthritis do not show any progression over five to 10 years. New research suggests that active mechanisms – not just aging and its accompanying processes – play a part in the development of osteoarthritis.

It is usually a simple matter to distinguish between osteoarthritis and rheumatoid arthritis. There are forms of osteoarthritis, however, that can look deceptively like rheumatoid arthritis. One such form is *erosive osteoarthritis*, in which the middle hand knuckle joints and/or the knuckles closest to the tips of the fingers often show bony enlargement. On X-rays, erosions are seen that can look very much like those seen in rheumatoid arthritis. The knuckles nearest the wrist are generally *not* involved in erosive osteoarthritis, which provides one way to distinguish this form of osteoarthritis from rheumatoid arthritis (see the image, this page). Furthermore, the wrists, elbows and ankles generally are not involved in erosive osteoarthritis, but are joints commonly affected in rheumatoid arthritis.

Occasionally, people develop osteoarthritis that is *symmetric* (affects the same joints on both sides of the body), which is a hallmark of rheumatoid arthritis. This may be seen primarily in both the hands, hips or knees.

Sometimes when a joint already has extensive damage from the inflammatory process of rheumatoid arthritis, but the inflammation itself is no longer present, the doctor may not be sure whether the damage was caused by osteoarthritis or rheumatoid arthritis. However, a detailed patient history and examination of other joints will usually allow the physician to determine the cause of the damage. At this point, the cause of damage is less important than addressing the damage itself (for instance, through the need for joint replacement surgery).

Fibromyalgia

Fibromyalgia is a syndrome that, like rheumatoid arthritis, is more common among women – about 90 percent of people with fibromyalgia are women, compared with 70 percent of people with rheumatoid arthritis. The most common symptom is widespread, generalized musculoskeletal pain, which may occur in the

back, shoulders, neck or any other part of the body. This widespread pain may raise a concern that the patient has rheumatoid arthritis, but there is no joint swelling or other evidence of inflammation in the joints seen in fibromyalgia.

People with fibromyalgia often have a history of sleep difficulties, and they may also experience problems in other organ systems – such as migraine headaches or irritable bowel syndrome. These are not associated with damage to the body, but can cause severe distress.

Although people with fibromyalgia may experience joint tenderness, tenderness is usually generalized to muscle groups. However, people with rheumatoid arthritis may also not have joint swelling at times

Disease Differences

Osteoarthritis	Rheumatoid Arthritis
Usually begins after age 40	Usually begins between ages 15 and 50
Usually develops slowly, over many years	May develop suddenly, within weeks or months
Affects a few joints and may occur on both sides of the body	Usually affects many joints, primarily the small joints on both sides of the body
Joint redness, warmth and swelling is usually minimal. Morning stiffness is common and may be severe but brief	Causes redness, warmth, swelling and prolonged morning stiffness of the joints
Affects only certain joints; most commonly hips, knees and lower back	Affects many joints; most commonly hands, wrists and feet
Doesn't cause a general feeling of sickness and fatigue	Often causes a general feeling of sickness and fatigue, as well as weight loss and fever

during the course of their disease, and they may show evidence of fibromyalgia. It appears that fibromyalgia is considerably more common in people with rheumatoid arthritis than in the general population – and in fact, some people have both rheumatoid arthritis and fibromyalgia. When this happens, both conditions may be mild, or one may be mild and the other severe.

It is important to distinguish whether rheumatoid arthritis or fibromyalgia may account for symptoms, because drugs used to treat rheumatoid arthritis usually do not help the symptoms that result from fibromyalgia. However, because many symptoms are common in both rheumatoid arthritis and fibromyalgia, including generalized muscle pain, morning stiffness, difficulty sleeping soundly and fatigue, the doctor and patient must sometimes make an educated guess about the likely cause of particular symptoms.

Gout

Gout has been called "the great masquerader" because it can mimic almost any other rheumatic disease. Gout occurs when an excess of *uric acid* in the body leads to the formation of crystals in the joint. The crystals can form deposits in joints, called tophi. These deposits can stimulate an inflammatory response that can cause an extremely painful attack of arthritis. Although gout most often occurs in the big toe, called *podagra,* it can involve virtually any joint or joints and, in time, the

attacks may become chronic and may resemble rheumatoid arthritis.

Certain features help distinguish gout from rheumatoid arthritis. First, gout usually occurs in men, whereas rheumatoid arthritis is more common in women. Second, gout usually does not involve the hands (at least in early disease), but rheumatoid arthritis does. Third, most pain and inflammation in gout occurs in episodes, rather than continually as in rheumatoid arthritis.

It is important to distinguish between gout and rheumatoid arthritis because specific medications that can lower uric acid levels and control gout attacks, differ from those used in treating rheumatoid arthritis.

Ankylosing Spondylitis

Ankylosing spondylitis is another generalized form of arthritis that can resemble rheumatoid arthritis. Joints commonly involved in ankylosing spondylitis are those of the back, neck, shoulders, hips and knees. Rheumatoid arthritis tends to affect the small joints of the hands and feet. As with gout, ankylosing spondylitis is thought to be more common among men, whereas rheumatoid arthritis is seen more often in women. Nevertheless, women also develop ankylosing spondylitis.

Although ankylosing spondylitis is a systemic disease like rheumatoid arthritis, it does not usually cause as much fatigue or poor sense of well-being.

The inflammation in ankylosing spondylitis occurs in the *enthesis,* or the place where the tendon inserts into the bone, as well as in the lining of the joint as seen in rheumatoid arthritis. People with ankylosing spondylitis tend to respond to different drugs, as well as different types of exercise programs, than those with RA, and these treatment differences reinforce the importance of a correct diagnosis.

Researchers have located a genetic marker (known as HLA-B27) that is associated with ankylosing spondylitis, reminiscent of the shared epitope of rheumatoid arthritis. However, this genetic marker is not a good diagnostic test for the disease because most people with the HLA-B27 marker do not have ankylosing spondylitis.

Some studies suggest that women with ankylosing spondylitis are more likely to experience signs of generalized inflammation – including more fatigue, poor sense of well-being and joint swelling – than men with ankylosing spondylitis.

Bursitis And Tendinitis

Bursitis and tendinitis are common conditions known as *soft tissue rheumatic syndromes*. Both conditions' symptoms include pain and inflammation in the structures and tissues around the joints. Bursitis is an irritation or inflammation of the *bursa*, a small sac located between bone and muscle, skin or tendon that allows for smooth movement between these structures. Tendinitis is an irritation or inflammation of the tendon, a cord that attaches muscle to bone. Bursitis and tendinitis can occur in many different joints in the body where bursae or tendons exist, including shoulders, elbows and hips.

The pain of bursitis and tendinitis are located near joints, so some people may mistake this pain for that of arthritis. But arthritis is the inflammation of the joint itself, not the structures around the joint.

Checkpoint: Your Diagnosis

Rheumatoid arthritis is not just the aches and pains of aging or of old injuries – it is a serious chronic illness that can affect many organs in your body. If you think you *may* have rheumatoid arthritis, you should see your doctor as soon as possible. Please remember that laboratory testing can be helpful, but does not provide the definitive information to make a diagnosis.

Not all doctors have extensive experience in the diagnosis and treatment of rheumatoid arthritis. Sometimes it is desirable to get a second opinion or to see a rheumatologist – a specialist in rheumatoid arthritis and related conditions. It is very important to control the joint inflammation of rheumatoid arthritis as early and as effectively as possible. Getting the right drug might reduce the chance of permanent damage and disability from rheumatoid arthritis.

Remember, you are the most important member of your health-care team, but you can't do it alone. Play it safe and see a doctor.

Sjögren's Syndrome

Sjögren's syndrome, which is also called sicca ("dry") syndrome, involves the salivary and lacrimal (tear-producing) glands, and leads to dry eyes and dry mouth. About 30 percent of people with rheumatoid arthritis have some evidence of Sjögren's syndrome.

Sjögren's syndrome is often diagnosed through a medical history and physical examination. Some doctors may also use any of a variety of tests. These tests may include a blood test to check the level of certain antibodies; tests to measure the dryness of eyes; a lip biopsy to examine the salivary glands; a salivary function test; or a urine test to check kidney function. Your doctor may send you to an ophthalmologist, an eye specialist, for an eye examination and to conduct some additional tests.

Sjögren's syndrome may be treated by a number of medications. Simple self-management strategies are also helpful, such as sipping water or chewing sugar-free gum or candies to temporarily ease dry mouth, and using over-the-counter lubricating eye drops to relieve dry eyes.

Felty's Syndrome

Felty's syndrome is a form of rheumatoid arthritis in which there is an enlargement of the spleen and a reduced number of white blood cells. Patients with Felty's syndrome are at increased risk for the development of infections. In some cases, it may be regarded (and treated) as a more severe form of rheumatoid arthritis.

Aggressive treatment with gold salts or methotrexate may be effective, even though

When Your Doctor Isn't Sure

Despite a medical history, physical examination and the appropriate tests, your doctor still isn't 100 percent sure whether you have rheumatoid arthritis or another type of inflammatory rheumatic disease. Should you worry?

You can probably relax. By tracking many people with inflammatory arthritis over the course of years, doctors have found that the most important matter is to identify and control the inflammation quickly. And the process for controlling inflammation is similar for most types of inflammatory arthritis, regardless of your specific diagnosis. For example, your doctor might try a nonsteroidal anti-inflammatory drug, a COX-2 specific inhibitor, or even low-dose corticosteroids (all of these drugs are discussed in detail in Chapter 11) over a period of one to two months, even when an exact diagnosis has not been established.

This initial treatment should make you feel a lot better, have less pain and function more easily – all to your benefit. The evidence suggests that as long as your joint inflammation is controlled, there is a low likelihood that you will develop joint damage.

they may not seem appropriate initially because they may reduce the white blood cell count. Sometimes surgical removal of the spleen is required to manage Felty's syndrome effectively.

Connective Tissue Diseases

A number of related diseases, referred to as connective tissue diseases, may be associated with arthritis, and can give the appearance of rheumatoid arthritis. Some of the more common forms of connective tissue disease are described below.

SYSTEMIC LUPUS ERYTHEMATOSUS (LUPUS)

Like rheumatoid arthritis, systemic lupus erythematosus (also called SLE or lupus) is characterized by musculoskeletal pain that is caused by inflammation and an autoimmune response. Almost all people with lupus will test positive for antinuclear antibodies (ANA), but up to one-half of those with rheumatoid arthritis also have a positive ANA test.

Arthritis and skin rashes are common in people with lupus. In addition, involvement of vital organs such as the kidney or brain may occur in lupus, leading to serious complications.

SCLERODERMA (SYSTEMIC SCLEROSIS)

This disease is characterized by tightening of the skin. People with scleroderma may experience a discoloration of the hands when exposed to cold (known as Raynaud's phenomenon). This may also be seen in people with rheumatoid arthritis. People with scleroderma may also have involvement of internal organs, in particular the lungs, kidneys and gastrointestinal track.

POLYMYOSITIS/DERMATOMYOSITIS

Polymyositis is a disease involving inflammation primarily in the muscles. This inflammation can lead to muscle weakness and permanent muscle damage. Some people with polymyositis develop rashes on their hands, face or trunk, a condition referred to as dermato("skin")myositis.

VASCULITIS

Vasculitis is an inflammation of the blood vessels that may affect any organ of the body. Some people with vasculitis may have arthritis that is difficult to distinguish from rheumatoid arthritis. In rare cases, someone with rheumatoid arthritis can develop a type of vasculitis called rheumatoid vasculitis, and it may be difficult to determine which one is the primary condition.

Chapter 6

More Than Joints:

When Other Body Parts Are Affected

Although rheumatoid arthritis most commonly affects your joints, it can also target other parts of your body, including organs you may not have expected to be involved in this disease. As we mentioned in Chapter 2, rheumatoid arthritis is called a systemic disease, meaning it involves the whole body. The swelling and pain in the joints and other parts of the body result from inflammation. Inflammation is a major reason you are likely to have an overall poor sense of well-being, with fatigue, fevers or weight loss during the course of the disease.

When examined carefully, many people with rheumatoid arthritis show some signs of disease affecting other organs, including the skin, eyes, mouth, lungs, heart, kidney, blood cells and spleen. Fortunately, such involvement is generally not severe, and doesn't produce any clinical symptoms. But sometimes, there can be important problems to address.

When other organs are affected in people with rheumatoid arthritis, an important consideration is whether the involvement is due to the disease itself, to side effects of the drugs used to treat rheumatoid arthritis, or to both.

Skin

Rheumatoid nodules are seen at some point in the disease in about one-half of people with rheumatoid arthritis. These nodules are actually lumps of tissue that form under the skin, often over bony areas exposed to pressure (such as on the fingers or around the elbow). No treatment is usually necessary, unless the nodule is located in a sensitive spot, such as where a person holds a pen. The nodules sometimes disappear on their own or with treatment. Interestingly, almost all people who develop these nodules also have rheumatoid factor, although doctors are unsure what (if any) the connection may be.

Drugs used to treat rheumatoid arthritis can also cause skin problems, such as rashes.

Blue or purplish bruises sometimes appear on the skin as a result of taking corticosteroids.

Some people with RA may be affected by vasculitis (inflammation of the blood vessels), which can cause red dots to appear on the skin. This is relatively unusual, but it may be a clue that the same process is occurring in internal organs such as the lungs or kidneys. Such involvement can have serious consequences if not brought under control, although aggressive treatment with corticosteroids, methotrexate and other *cytotoxic* drugs (chemicals that destroy cells or prevent their multiplication) usually resolves the problem.

Eyes

People with rheumatoid arthritis who also have Sjögren's syndrome, which was mentioned in the last chapter, may experience dry eyes. The problem of dry eyes may be treated by the use of "artificial tears" eye drops. In severe cases, a special surgical procedure may help lubricate the eyes.

Some people with rheumatoid arthritis may also have an inflammation of the eyes known as *scleritis*. Doctors may treat scleritis with eye drops, as well as aggressive anti-inflammatory medications. A rare complication of scleritis is *scleromalacia perforans*, in which the eye can be permanently damaged by severe inflammation. If you have rheumatoid arthritis and develop eye redness that persists longer than a few days, seek examination by an eye-care professional, such as an ophthalmologist, to determine if you need special treatment for scleritis. However, let's emphasize that severe eye inflammation is rare – most people with RA will not experience this condition.

To Treat Aggressively or To Back Off – That's the Quest

The drugs used to treat rheumatoid arthritis, which are explored in depth in Chapter 11, are powerful. That is one reason doctors carefully monitor their patients for possible side effects. However, one problem in rheumatoid arthritis is to determine whether the complication is an effect of the disease process, in which the body's own immune system seemingly turns against itself, or if a drug is causing the problem.

This is where the dilemma occurs: When possible side effects are noted, the tendency is to back off from aggressive treatment by reducing dosages or stopping drugs altogether. However, in some people this approach may be a mistake.

If you face a similar situation, talk to your doctor about your options. It should always be a consideration that organ involvement in some (but certainly not all) people with rheumatoid arthritis may more likely be a component of the disease than a side effect of treatment. The problem should continue to be treated aggressively with the appropriate drugs.

Mouth

In addition to dry eyes, people with Sjögren's syndrome may experience a severely dry mouth, because of a decrease in the body's production of saliva. People with Sjögren's syndrome should drink plenty of fluids to keep the mouth moist. Good dental hygiene is a must, as bacteria tend to flourish without the usual flow of saliva in the mouth. Oral medications exist to help people treat the dryness of Sjögren's syndrome.

Mouth sores or oral ulcers are a frequent complication of treatment with methotrexate, and sometimes with injectable gold. Mouthwashes and lower methotrexate doses can often alleviate the problem.

Personally Speaking   Stories from real people with rheumatoid arthritis

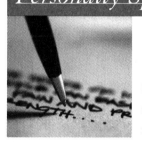

"**M**y day is very much like anyone else's day. I am a social worker and I work full time. It's hard to get out of bed on some mornings. My hands and ankles are almost always stiff. It's hard to work buttons and zippers first thing in the morning, and if my ankles are swollen, I have to pick shoes that will fit on my feet. As I dress myself though, I start to loosen up and by the time I have my makeup on and leave for work, I'm able to move pretty well.

Working with RA: Daily Challenges
by Dawn Maria Dent, Philadelphia, PA

"My workday is never the same. On days when my hands are sore, I generally stay away from typing and make phone calls and file papers instead. Some days I have to go in the field, and might have to drive long distances. Driving isn't easy when my hands and ankles hurt. When I'm not feeling well, I get tired easily and it's hard to make it through the day. I'm especially tired the morning after I take my methotrexate. It would be very easy to stay home whenever I didn't feel well, and I think if I started to do that I would be home pretty often. Without my job I would never be able to afford my medical bills.

"It's hard to tell people how you feel when you don't feel well. Some people try to tell me that if I exercised more or changed my diet, my RA would go away. Even though I keep myself active and do as much as I can, there are times when I just can't do any more, and not everyone realizes that the pain isn't something you can just work through or talk yourself out of. Most of the people in my life treat me the same as they always did. I don't expect any extra help because I have RA. I know that if I were at the stage I'm at now and didn't have the treatments that are available today I wouldn't be able to function nearly as well as I do. I don't expect people to understand what I'm going through, I just expect them to be patient with me when I'm not feeling well."

Lungs

Rheumatoid arthritis can also affect the lungs, including an inflammation of the lining of the lungs known as *pleurisy.* Pleurisy can cause pain when taking a deep breath. Standard anti-inflammatory treatments for rheumatoid arthritis can alleviate this inflammation. Occasionally, people with rheumatoid arthritis may develop scarring, called *pulmonary fibrosis,* which leads to progressive shortness of breath.

Methotrexate, one of the most common RA treatments, can sometimes cause a complication known as "methotrexate lung" or "methotrexate pneumonia." The pneumonia generally goes away when the methotrexate is stopped. Most people can safely resume taking methotrexate a few weeks after an episode of methotrexate pneumonia. Similar drug-induced pneumonias have also been reported with other, less common drugs used to treat rheumatoid arthritis, including injectable gold and penicillamine.

Sometimes it's difficult for your doctor to tell whether a lung problem results from rheumatoid arthritis or from a drug. In such cases, you and your doctor may consider other diagnostic testing. This is another example of how RA and its treatments must be monitored over time.

Heart

Occasionally, people with rheumatoid arthritis may develop *pericarditis* (inflammation of the lining surrounding the heart), leading to chest pain or discomfort and requiring direct treatment.

Kidneys

Kidneys remove waste products from the body. In some people with rheumatoid arthritis, kidney function (as measured by levels of blood urea nitrogen [BUN] or creatinine) may be reduced. Kidney problems are more likely related to side effects of RA drugs – such as cyclosporine (*Neoral*) or a nonsteroidal anti-inflammatory drug (NSAID) – than to the disease itself. If you are taking one of these drugs, your doctor will monitor your renal (kidney) function at periodic intervals to watch for problems.

Blood-Forming Cells

People with rheumatoid arthritis may experience a particular type of *anemia,* or reduction in the number of red blood cells. No special treatment is necessary for this condition, which improves as the level of inflammation in the body is brought under control.

Occasionally, people with RA develop *iron-deficiency anemia,* treated by iron replacement supplements. *Pernicious anemia,* relatively rare, can be corrected with vitamin B12 injections and/or folic acid. People with Felty's syndrome can experience a decrease in white blood cells due to enlargement of the spleen, something treated by either drugs or, in some cases, removal of the spleen.

People with very active inflammation may have high levels of blood platelets; these levels return toward normal when the inflammation is controlled. Aggressive drug treatment of rheumatoid arthritis may cause decreased numbers of platelets, a condition called *thrombocytopenia,* if the bone marrow is suppressed. Some drugs may cause a decrease in white blood cells. Regular monitoring will identify these problems so they may be treated.

Spleen

Felty's syndrome occurs when people with rheumatoid arthritis have a reduced number of white blood cells and an enlarged spleen. Some doctors consider this syndrome to be linked to a more severe form of rheumatoid arthritis. Treatments should be aggressive. There appears to be an increased rise of non-Hodgkin's lymphoma in people with rheumatoid arthritis who develop Felty's syndrome.

As you've learned, rheumatoid arthritis can affect many different parts of the body and in many different ways. Regular monitoring by your physician is important, and following the treatment plan outlined by your physician will help alleviate many problems. But what can you expect long-term from RA? In the next chapter, we'll examine long-term prognosis and how new approaches to treatment are improving that prognosis.

Chapter 7

The Long Haul:

What To Expect With RA Over Time

Chronic diseases like rheumatoid arthritis are, by definition, long-lasting. Therefore, you may be as concerned with what will happen to you years from now as you are with what is happening in your body today. That's completely understandable, especially with rheumatoid arthritis. Living with RA can be very frustrating. You may experience periods of flare and periods of seeming remission, times when your joints are stiff and painful and times when you feel fine. It's hard to know what to expect on a day-to-day basis and tough to plan ahead.

If you know other people with rheumatoid arthritis, you may be even more confused. You may meet one person with a case of RA that is quite severe, causing her to quit working. You might meet another person who is able to continue working and to be involved in various physical activities. You might worry about what outcome you will experience.

All people with rheumatoid arthritis are individuals, so it's practically impossible to predict exactly how anyone's disease will progress over time. Nonetheless, there are some general guidelines that can help you and your doctor establish a reasonable possibility of what might happen over the course of this chronic disease.

Making a Prediction – Some General Guidelines

Some clues that can help determine the long-term course and severity of rheumatoid arthritis cannot be influenced by you – such as the number of joints that are involved or the level of C-reactive protein (CRP) in the blood. However, there are other clues that you *can* affect, such as how quickly treatment is started and how well you can adapt to the challenges of dealing with rheumatoid arthritis. These general guidelines about your long-term outcome include the following:

• **The actual rate of progression of the disease.** This is what some people call the "natural history" or the course that the disease takes in your body. Careful monitoring over the course of several months is often the most helpful method to predict the course of disease. A combination of factors may determine the rate of progression, including the level of pain, fatigue, tenderness and swelling; level of function and disability; and counting the number of involved joints. Lab tests may provide more information.

• **How quickly treatment is begun.** When you first notice signs of rheumatoid arthritis, get a proper diagnosis. We cannot stress enough how important this is. The sooner treatment is started (and treatment, in almost all cases, will involve drugs that can only be prescribed by a doctor), the sooner your inflammation can be brought under control. Chronic, untreated inflammation can lead to permanent, long-term damage to the joints, so get a doctor's diagnosis as quickly as possible.

• **How aggressively the disease is treated.** Early, aggressive treatment is the best tactic in fighting RA. Medications should be strong enough to bring the inflammation under control, not just to reduce the symptoms, as early as possible. Reducing symptoms may reduce the underlying damage being caused to the joints, and may make you feel better, but it's important to use aggressive treatment to prevent long-term joint damage too.

• **How the individual is coping with the disease.** People who feel they are in control of their chronic disease tend to have a

better long-term outlook. We call this type of coping *self-efficacy*, and this concept is the cornerstone of this book. Self-efficacy in rheumatoid arthritis includes using joint-protection techniques, exercising, following your treatment plan and keeping a positive outlook.

Another Clue: Your Disease Type

It's difficult to predict the course of your disease when you have rheumatoid arthritis, as each case is unique in its progression. Some may find that their disease subsides after a few months, while others turn out to have a disease course with inflammation and joint involvement that seems to get worse over time (especially if not treated). Still others seem to travel a middle road, their disease well controlled by medications (see box, p. 47). Let's discuss the three main types of rheumatoid arthritis, so you can better understand where your case may fall and what prognosis you may expect.

TYPE I DISEASE

In the late 1960s, large studies involving the entire population of certain areas were conducted to see how many people might meet the criteria for rheumatoid arthritis. As it turned out, about two percent of the population met these criteria. About 75 percent of those who met the criteria did not show evidence of having rheumatoid arthritis three to five years later. Among those who initially met the criteria for RA but did not have evidence of having the disease after five

The Three Types of Rheumatoid Arthritis			
	TYPE I	TYPE II	TYPE III
Progression	Spontaneous remission	Minimal disease progress	Serious disease progress
Percentage of people with type	5-20%	5-20%	60-90%
How is it distinguished?	Neg. rheumatoid factor	Lasts more than six months, positive lab findings	Lasts more than six months, positive lab findings
Also called	Inflammatory arthritis, reactive arthritis, post-viral arthritis	Mild rheumatoid arthritis	Progressive inflammatory symmetrical arthritis

years, apparently many never saw a doctor about their symptoms.

It now seems likely that if a person has symptoms that meet the criteria for rheumatoid arthritis for less than six months, there is a good chance that the condition will go away on its own. Doctors now better understand the early stages of RA and can better recognize this Type I disease form of rheumatoid arthritis that does not tend to progress. In fact, they may call it something other than rheumatoid arthritis – perhaps inflammatory polyarthritis. The term rheumatoid arthritis is now usually reserved for a more severe case of the disease.

TYPE II DISEASE

Most people who meet the criteria for rheumatoid arthritis and have experienced arthritis in symmetrical joints – that is, both wrists, both hands and so on – for longer than six months do not experience a spontaneous remission of their symptoms. A minority of these people with progressive rheumatoid arthritis, from five percent to 20 percent, may have a mild disease course that can be controlled with less aggressive therapy, such as nonsteroidal anti-inflammatory drugs (NSAIDs) alone. This form of rheumatoid arthritis is referred to as Type II disease. Although Type II disease is progressive, it tends to cause less severe damage to joints and often does not affect other parts of the body.

TYPE III DISEASE OR PISA

Most people who have symptoms of rheumatoid arthritis for longer than six months will have what is known as persistent inflammatory symmetrical arthritis (PISA) or Type III disease. This is the most severe type of RA, affecting 60 percent to 90 percent of people whose disease is monitored by a doctor. The symptoms usually cannot be controlled with NSAIDs alone. Usually, stronger disease-modifying antirheumatic drugs (known as DMARDs, see Chapter 11) are needed as well to control inflammation and prevent damage.

Yes, Type III rheumatoid arthritis can have long-term consequences and mean years of taking medications and being monitored regularly by a physician. However, new developments in treatment lead us to re-examine the prognosis for people with Type III RA. New information, new drugs and more aggressive treatment strategies now greatly improve the long-term outlook for this population. Because of these advances and others that are just on the horizon, doctors believe that the sort of joint damage that was common 20 years ago will soon be considered a thing of the past. People with RA now have more treatment options, with fewer side effects, than ever before.

Why It's Important To See a Doctor

It's clear that the first six months that you experience RA symptoms are key. In some cases, the disease may go away on its own. In others, it may progress and lead to permanent damage. Why, then, is it important to see a doctor as quickly as possible if you think you may have rheumatoid arthritis?

Can't you just wait it out and see if it gets better on its own?

First, it's important to see a doctor to make sure that you actually have rheumatoid arthritis, and not another disease, as mentioned in Chapter 4. An experienced doctor will consider all the evidence and make a diagnosis. Only an accurate diagnosis can assure you that you are taking the proper treatments for your condition.

Second, you should establish some benchmark measurements during the early months of your disease to track its progression. In these early months, your doctor will look for persistent joint swelling, rheumatoid factor and even early evidence of changes on X-rays.

Third, if your doctor notices evidence of progressive disease during an early visit, he or she will begin treatment to control inflammation. These drug treatments can prevent damage to joints down the line. New and effective drugs, with fewer side effects than past drugs, can help avoid serious problems and greatly improve the long-term outlook with rheumatoid arthritis.

Finally, there's nothing wrong with seeing your doctor about a condition that may get better on its own. In fact, about one half of all visits to physicians involve such situations. In this case, it's truly better to be safe than sorry!

What Changes You Can Expect

During the 1980s, doctors realized that the treatment approaches for rheumatoid arthritis at the time did not provide a positive long-term outlook for their patients. Several rheumatology centers reported that most people with rheumatoid arthritis experienced extensive joint damage, apparent in the progression of their X-rays, severe declines in ability to function, frequent work disability, and even shortened life span. Something had to change. Those observations led to renewed efforts to treat rheumatoid arthritis more effectively, and the last 10 years has seen dramatic change in treatment options and approaches.

Doctors now have a different outlook on how rheumatoid arthritis should progress, and they monitor the progression of their patients' disease through various tests and observations. Let's review how they review changes in patients' progress now.

X-RAY CHANGES

Over time, X-rays show joint damage in almost all people with rheumatoid arthritis who are untreated or who are not receiving aggressive treatment to control the disease. In fact, about seven of 10 people who have rheumatoid arthritis develop joint changes that can be seen on X-rays within two years. A magnetic resonance imaging (MRI) scan may show damage to joints even earlier.

Although new medications can now reduce the chances of joint damage, once it occurs, it's usually irreversible. (Surgical replacement of a joint may be the only treatment option at that point, and this option is not appropriate in every case. Surgery will be discussed further in Chapter 12.) In most people, the most rapid damage occurs early

Personally Speaking Stories from real people with rheumatoid arthritis

"I am a registered nurse. I have had rheumatoid arthritis for several years with the usual symptoms of joint pain and swelling. I had rheumatic fever as a child.

"Approximately five years ago, I started having severe vertigo. It was so severe, I went to the emergency room with the assistance of a friend, and I had severe vomiting and was literally not able to stand. All the usual tests were run, and I was given anti-nausea treatments.

Multiple Complications: A Nurse Speaks Out
by Judith Nave, Anderson, IN

"I was better after approximately one year. Then I started losing my sight in my right eye. After one year, I was totally blind in my right eye and referred to a university medical center. To make a long story short, I had arthritis affecting my right eye. And after the fact, they concluded I had rheumatoid arthritis that was also affecting my right inner ear. I am nearly blind in my right eye, but have some vision with a contact lens. I didn't realize rheumatoid arthritis could do that to you."

on, when inflammation is present. This is yet another reason for you to get a diagnosis and begin drug treatment.

CHANGES IN FUNCTION

Doctors will also measure the progress of rheumatoid arthritis by observing your ability to perform ordinary tasks, such as dressing, reaching, walking or operating household tools. Overall, more than 90 percent of people with rheumatoid arthritis report having some problems in doing their usual activities. Loss of function occurs most rapidly during the first few years of the disease.

Now that treatment is more aggressive, health-care professionals have a new understanding of the biopsychosocial approach to treatment (see Chapter 1) and people with rheumatoid arthritis are more involved in managing their arthritis, so the percentage of people with RA who report serious loss of function has come down. The sooner you learn to adapt your movements or to use special aids to help you do various tasks, the sooner you will regain your freedom and ability to work and take care of yourself.

How do you cope with losing dexterity and the ability to do basic tasks? You might seek help from family members or coworkers, use special aids or devices (such as special door handle attachments), or even plan ahead to avoid excessive activity. Being creative, and adapting your surroundings and activities, can have a positive impact. More specific strategies will be discussed later in the book.

WORK DISABILITY

One of the more serious possible consequences of rheumatoid arthritis is work disability. Some figures show that more than one half of people with rheumatoid arthritis become unable to work after 10 years. This translates into almost one million people in the United States alone who may experience work disability because of this disease. That's a serious economic problem. Yet new treatments for RA may improve your outlook for staying on the job.

Interestingly, the severity of disease does not accurately predict who will become disabled from work. Complex factors determine whether a person becomes unable to work, including the person's age, occupation, employer and the amount of control the person has over the pace of his or her job.

A number of resources are available to help people with disabilities continue to work (see sidebar, next page). Since the passage of the Americans with Disabilities Act (ADA) in 1990, most employers are required by law to provide reasonable accommodations to help their employees keep working. For example, if you must stand all day to supervise employees, you may ask for job modifications from your employer.

You may be concerned about whether you can continue working. Remember, this choice should be made only after you have explored all the alternatives carefully, both with your doctor and with your employer. Many job modifications cost little and can allow you to keep working without exhausting yourself or putting pressure on your joints. Many employers now allow teleworking and other alternatives to working on-site every day. While your health condition is a personal and private matter, you may need to discuss your diagnosis with your employer at some point to acquire modifications or a revised work schedule. The Arthritis Foundation offers free

If You Face Work Disability

While many people with rheumatoid arthritis continue to work – sometimes with modifications to workspaces, schedules or even jobs – some do face the real possibility of having to go on work disability. Helpful resources are available if you find that you are facing this choice. Career counseling and vocational testing services of the state-federal vocational rehabilitation program are available at no cost and are located in all 50 states. These and some other resources are listed below.

GOVERNMENT-SPONSORED VOCATIONAL REHABILITATION SERVICES

Most people with rheumatoid arthritis should be eligible for the following services: vocational counseling and testing; job placement; assistance with resume preparation and interview skills; payment for job accommodations, training, education and travel. Check your local government listings or websites to find more information on vocational services in your area. Or, check the website of the U.S. Department of Labor, www.dol.gov, for more information on general rights and services.

INDEPENDENT LIVING CENTERS

These centers provide advocacy services and programs that enable people with disabilities to live on their own. For more information, go to the website of Independent Living Research Utilization, a program of the Institute for Rehabilitation and Research, at www.ilru.org.

JOB ACCOMMODATION NETWORK

This free consulting service, operated by the President's Committee on Employment of People with Disabilities, provides information about the Americans with Disabilities Act and types of job accommodations. (800) 526-7234 or www.dol.gov.

DISABILITY AND BUSINESS TECHNICAL ASSISTANCE CENTERS

Centers are available in each region of the country to advise businesses and individuals about accommodations. (800) 949-4232.

THE ARTHRITIS FOUNDATION

The Arthritis Foundation has free publications on employment challenges for people with arthritis, including *Arthritis and the Workplace* and *Take Charge: Money Matters and Your Arthritis*. Order your free copy by calling (800) 283-7800 or logging on to www.arthritis.org.

publications to help you and your employer better understand the challenges you face. Call (800) 283-7800 or log on to www.arthritis.org to get your copy.

LIFE SPAN

People with rheumatoid arthritis experience many health conditions more often than the average population: infections, pulmonary disease, renal disease and gastrointestinal problems, to name a few. In addition, studies show that severe rheumatoid arthritis may decrease a person's life span by as much as 10 to 15 years compared to someone without the disease. However, many factors can determine how RA affects life span, including age of onset, the number of involved joints and ability to carry out daily activities, among others. Your approach to life with rheumatoid arthritis can have a positive impact, including taking care of your general health, not smoking, following your doctor's instructions, eating a healthy diet, getting exercise, and other good habits.

In the past five years, a number of innovative, highly effective treatments (which will be discussed fully in Chapter 11) for RA became available. These treatments can reduce serious complications and enhance the life span – as well as the quality of life – of people with rheumatoid arthritis. So the outlook now is much better than ever before.

Part Two

Medical Management:
What to Expect

Chapter 8

Keeping Tabs:
Evaluating and Monitoring Your Rheumatoid Arthritis

So far, we've learned that getting a proper diagnosis of your rheumatoid arthritis is the first, most important step. Because RA is chronic and may change over time, it's equally important to get regular monitoring to evaluate the progress of your disease over time, as well as to check on the effectiveness of your treatments. The goal of these treatments should be to control your symptoms as much as possible and to prevent permanent joint damage.

Rheumatologists measure rheumatoid arthritis disease activity in their patients through different methods, so they can determine the best individual treatment plan for each person. Even though RA varies from person to person, there are certain guidelines that doctors use to discover how well current treatments are working, or whether an additional or alternative drug is needed.

Tests and measures that doctors used to diagnose the disease in the first place are also used for ongoing evaluation and monitoring. For example, a doctor may examine a patient's joints to quickly determine the extent of joint swelling, tenderness and range of motion, as well as how many joints are involved. In addition, X-rays, laboratory tests, functional measures and patient questionnaires all provide valuable information. Patient questionnaires, which allow the person living with the disease to describe his or her own symptoms and feel-ings, are an especially rich source of information on pain, fatigue, basic functioning, psychological distress and other consequences of rheumatoid arthritis.

Let's look at some of the methods and measures used to evaluate disease activity over time, as well as to monitor your drugs' effectiveness and possible adverse effects. Although there are many different ways to evaluate and monitor rheumatoid arthritis, it is possible to group these measures into three fairly broad categories.

- **Measures of inflammatory activity.** Doctors measure joint tenderness and swelling, as well as administer laboratory tests like sedimentation rate and C-reactive protein tests, in order to measure inflammatory activity in the joints. These measures are most useful in the first few years of rheumatoid arthritis, when severe inflammation is usually present, without any joint damage. These measures can change over time to show whether your current drug treatments are effectively reducing your inflammation.
- **Measures of damage.** Doctors assess joint damage through examinations of your mobility and joint alignment, as well as through X-rays and specialized tests of function, such as walk times or button tests. Long-term joint damage is one of the more worrisome aspects of rheumatoid arthritis. These measures help your doctor evaluate your quality of life, because joint damage in part determines a person's ability to carry out daily activities. Measures of damage mostly assess changes over months to years.
- **Measures of outcome.** The biggest concern for a person with RA is: How will this disease affect me, particularly long-term? You're concerned with loss of function, work disability, joint destruction and financial costs associated with the disease. Experts who study the entire rheumatoid arthritis population can predict average outcomes of people with RA through long-term studies (studies that follow a group of individuals over the course of many years),

or by sifting through information such as applications for disability related to rheumatoid arthritis. This general information may be of use to you as an individual, by telling you what you may expect. But your doctor can tell you more specific information based on your unique situation, and give you advice on how to improve your outcome through treatments or lifestyle modifications.

These three types of measures do not necessarily measure the same thing. For example, joint tenderness is a very effective measure of disease activity, but it is not meaningfully associated with changes that show up on X-rays. Although this may be hard to understand, it is important. Rheumatologists have had serious concerns over the last 15 years as evidence shows that, in some cases, measures of inflammatory activity may be stable while joint and organ damage still progresses. This problem emerged as people were treated under a more cautious, less aggressive approach. The new approach to treatment – aggressive, early treatment of inflammation – may alleviate this problem.

Joint Examinations

Joint examination is one of the key ways to evaluate RA disease activity. Changes in your joint count, or the number of joints that are tender or swollen, measure the inflammation associated with rheumatoid arthritis. Joint counts help your doctor track disease progression or improvement. In addition, your doctor will probably look for any pain during motion, limitation in the motion of your joint or joint malalignment. When the structures in the joint fail to align properly, joint function is hampered.

There are several different methods used for joint counts, ranging from the simple (a rating or normal or abnormal for each joint) to the complex (four or more possible gradations for each joint). Simpler measures perform just as well as the more complex ones, and they are easier to use. The number of joints that are counted also varies, from as few as 28 to as many as 70. In long-term studies, joint counts have proved quite useful in assessing, monitoring and even predicting the course of rheumatoid arthritis.

Personally Speaking — Stories from real people with rheumatoid arthritis

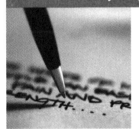

RA Challenges: Seeking Information and Staying Active
by Jaimie Walton,
Tulsa, OK

"I developed joint pain, specifically in my feet, toes, knees, hands and fingers, in early November 2003. I was an ER nurse and I can no longer work at bedside nursing. I believed my joint pain was nothing and would go away. It worsened and I went to see a rheumatologist. X-rays were done which showed changes related to RA. I also have problems with my urinary system and my eyes.

"I've had many difficulties. Opening doors, opening tops of containers, opening a can of soda – all of these things have become chores. When I go shopping, I have a lot of pain when I need to squat to get something on a lower shelf. My husband has to help me up because my knees are so painful. I had to purchase a larger size shoe, and I bought ones that slip on so I don't have to tie them. I am unable to complete the blanket I was crocheting for my daughter.

"There are days when I cry because I don't know who to talk to or what to do. When I have very bad days, my husband comes home for lunch to help me. At 42, I feel like I have done something wrong and I'm being punished. Some days the pain is so bad, I just sit and cry. I try to keep moving. I can't lift much nor can I walk far. I go to the gym and try to swim, and I will be starting a water-exercise program to help keep the joints moving without stress. I try to walk my dog around the block every day, which helps both of us.

"I read all information about RA. I read what others with RA have to say about their lives. I will accept advice from anyone who can help me and I will try anything that has worked for someone else if I can."

X-rays and Other Imaging Techniques

X-rays (also called *radiographs*) are useful for showing specific types of changes associated with rheumatoid arthritis. Doctors can detect narrowing of the joint space, erosion of the structures in the joint and malalignment of the joint itself. In addition, X-rays can show changes of osteoporosis, or thinning of the bones. This condition can be very serious and lead to painful, debilitating fractures. People with rheumatoid arthritis may be at higher risk of developing osteoporosis, and some drugs used to treat rheumatoid arthritis, such as corticosteroids, can also increase your risk.

X-rays are useful for evaluating joint damage. Sometimes your doctor will take what are known as "baseline X-rays" when you are first diagnosed with rheumatoid arthritis. These are used as a basis for comparison through the years so that any changes are more easily noted.

Other, more advanced imaging techniques, such as magnetic resonance imaging (MRI) and ultrasound scanning, help doctors find evidence of inflammation before joint damage occurs. X-rays are less sensitive and primarily assess damaged joints. These newer imaging techniques may be used more often in the future for evaluating and monitoring disease activity.

Laboratory Tests

The two most widely used laboratory tests to assess inflammation are the erythrocyte sedimentation rate (ESR or sed rate), and C-reactive protein (CRP). As we noted before, these tests are not always abnormal in people with rheumatoid arthritis – only 60 percent to 70 percent of people with the disease show elevated levels of these measures. However, in people who do have elevated levels, the ESR and CRP can provide valuable information about disease activity over time.

Blood counts often are used to monitor for adverse side effects of medications used to treat rheumatoid arthritis, such as methotrexate. These tests may be repeated periodically. For example, a low white blood cell count can indicate suppression of blood cell formation in the bone marrow. Low red blood cell counts suggest anemia, and can be caused by small amounts of bleeding in the gastrointestinal tract when taking certain drugs such as nonsteroidal anti-inflammatory drugs (NSAIDs).

A urinalysis, a test done on a sample of urine to determine its contents, may also be used periodically to see whether your urine contains red blood cells, protein or a variety of other abnormal substances. Again, these measures are used to monitor the effects of strong medications.

Liver function tests measure the levels of enzymes produced by the liver. The level may be elevated in people taking certain drugs for rheumatoid arthritis, including methotrexate and leflunomide (*Arava*). The tests are usually repeated every four to eight weeks for individuals using these drugs, and the results are closely monitored.

Physical Function Measures

Physical measures of function may indicate both inflammatory activity and evidence of long-term joint damage. These measures (discussed in Chapter 3) may be repeated for comparison from one visit to another. Some of the more commonly used include measures of grip strength, walking time and manual dexterity (button test and others).

Self-Report Questionnaires

Self-report questionnaires provide a way to measure symptoms and concerns that are difficult to quantify by other, more medical methods such as laboratory tests or X-rays.

They may ask questions about pain, fatigue, loss in functional status and psychological distress. Patients can provide the best information about improvements or worsening in these areas. As with other evaluative measures, doctors usually repeat questionnaires regularly to keep track of important data.

Patient questionnaires provide another avenue for your input, by asking for information that only you can provide. Take the time to fill out these questionnaires as completely, accurately and honestly as possible. Work with your doctor and other health-care professionals to develop the best treatment plan and help evaluate its effectiveness over time.

Chapter 9

Your Health-Care Team:

Get To Know Your Key Players

Now we have explored what rheumatoid arthritis is and how it can affect your body. Let's delve into some of the keys to the medical management of rheumatoid arthritis: What does it involve and how can you participate to get the best care and treatment possible?

Most people think of "medical management" in terms of drugs or medications prescribed by a doctor. You may feel that as a patient, you are a passive participant in the process. That isn't true! You are a very important player in this game – in fact, you are the manager of a "health-care team," a collection of talented, important people who all play a position in your overall treatment. In a chronic disease like rheumatoid arthritis, you and your health-care team can work together to do a great deal to help manage the effects of the disease.

In this chapter, we discuss the health-care professionals on your team. You may not have all of these players on your particular roster, but it's important to know what these various professionals do in case you do need to seek their care. In Chapter 10, we'll discuss self-management in more detail to illustrate what you can do to improve your outlook with rheumatoid arthritis. In Chapter 11, we'll review the various drugs you may take to treat your disease and its symptoms.

Who's on Your Health-Care Team?

Yes, you and your primary doctor should form a partnership in managing your arthritis. For most people with rheumatoid arthritis, that doctor is a rheumatologist. But he or she may only be one of the health-care professionals you consult for your care at various points in the course of your disease.

Like the disease itself, your individual needs may vary when it comes to your health-care team. Some people do well working with only their rheumatologist and his or her office staff, including nurses, nurse practitioners and physician assistants, depending on the practice. Other people turn to many other health-care professionals or therapists to be involved in their care.

To use an old metaphor, think of your arthritis care in terms of a play to be staged. The play should not be a "one-man show," nor should it be a cast of thousands. Instead, envision it as an ensemble production, in which each player has a very particular and necessary role. In some acts, only two or three players will appear; in others, the whole cast may be on stage. Finally, you need to view yourself as not only playing a key part, but being the director as well. It will be up to you to decide which players can be used most effectively in which scenes.

Meet the Players

The players on your health-care team depend on the particular problems or symptoms you encounter, your ability to cope with your disease and its effects, your insurance coverage, and the availability of services in your area. The following is a list and brief description of some of the health-care professionals who may play a role in your treatment.

DOCTORS

When we refer to doctors or physicians here, we refer to medical professionals with a medical doctor (MD) degree and level of training, or in some cases, a doctor of osteopathy (DO) degree. There are other medical professionals, such as doctors of podiatric medicine (DPM) and others, that can also be included in the general category

of "doctors," although they specialize in certain types of care and don't provide general medical care. Doctors should fall into two subcategories: primary-care physicians, who provide general care, and specialists (or subspecialists), who undergo additional years of training in a specific area of medical care.

Family physicians, general practitioners and *primary-care physicians* provide medical care for adults and children with different types of arthritis and related conditions. These doctors provide the cornerstone of medical treatment for your general health, and manage common additional medical problems such as high blood pressure or gastrointestinal distress. These general doctors can also help you locate a specialist. Every person should have a family physician or internist as a primary-care doctor – a specialist should not be your only doctor.

Internists specialize in internal medicine and treating adult diseases. They may be general internists who act as primary-care physicians, or they may be subspecialists who have completed additional training in specific types of disease. A general internist provides general care to adults and often helps select subspecialists. Internists should not be confused with *interns*, who are doctors doing a year's training in a hospital after graduating from medical school.

Rheumatologists are internists who have further training to treat people with arthritis or related diseases that affect the joints, muscles, bones, skin and other tissues. Most people with rheumatoid arthritis are referred to a rheumatologist at least at some point in their care for special assessment and treatment. Some rheumatologists may also have training in pediatrics, orthopaedics, physical medicine, sports medicine or other medical fields.

Orthopaedic surgeons or *orthopaedists* are doctors who specialize in diseases of the bone. The general area of care for specialists in orthopaedics involves mechanical problems of bones and joints, in contrast to inflammatory problems such as rheumatoid arthritis. Orthopaedists are the doctors who set fractures, repair or replace a damaged hip, knee or other joint, and treat other bone ailments. Many orthopaedists subspecialize in particular areas, such as hand surgery, sports medicine, joint replacement, etc.

When a person develops musculoskeletal pain, it is often not clear whether the problem is mechanical, inflammatory, or even based on some other type of cause, such as an infection or metabolic problem. Therefore, people with rheumatoid arthritis may be referred at first to an orthopaedic surgeon.

Pediatricians treat childhood diseases. A child who develops arthritis will see a pediatrician at first. Certain pediatricians known as *pediatric rheumatologists* specialize in the care of arthritis in children. These specialist pediatricians are usually located only in large cities or medical centers. A visit to such a specialist can be extremely helpful to a child with juvenile arthritis and is recommended if possible.

Personally Speaking   Stories from real people with rheumatoid arthritis

"**L**ife is not so beautiful for my mother, Kathy, at times. She has been recently diagnosed with rheumatoid arthritis, and it's slowly beginning to cripple her life. She has so much pain in her knees and arms and hands. It breaks my heart to see her in

My Mother's RA: An Inspiration
by Gabrielle Rogers, Garland, TX

pain. She fears that she will be confined to a wheelchair and be deformed. If I were she, I'd fear the same things. Nevertheless, she is strong. She still manages to raise four children and work and be an excellent mom, but the pain can be so overwhelming for her.

"She means so much to me. She and my father adopted me when I was an infant. I don't want her to suffer like this. Though it may seem hopeless to relieve pain and swelling at times, she has never ever pointed the finger at God. Even in the midst of pain she gives God thanks and praise – that is a true survivor. I hope that she will one day soon get the medicine needed to stop this pain she has and to help her live an easier life. But even so, she is an inspiration to me daily."

Physiatrists are doctors who direct physical therapy and rehabilitation programs. Comprehensive rehabilitation programs may have been more common 10 or 20 years ago when joint destruction was seen in most people with rheumatoid arthritis. Inflammation is better controlled at this time, and this type of treatment may be less necessary in general for people with rheumatoid arthritis. However, physical therapy still plays a major role in treatment for some people with rheumatoid arthritis.

Podiatrists or *chiropodists* are doctors with particular training in the care of the feet. These doctors may be extremely helpful to certain people with extensive disease involvement of their feet.

Psychiatrists are medical doctors who treat mental or emotional problems that need special attention. They can prescribe medications for treating the problems.

Psychologists are also trained to treat mental or emotional problems, but have a doctor of philosophy (PhD) rather than a medical degree (MD) and therefore do not prescribe medications. Psychiatrists and psychologists can be very helpful to people who have rheumatoid arthritis, as it is not uncommon that psychological issues affect their daily lives.

OTHER HEALTH-CARE PROFESSIONALS

Some *nurses* and *nurse practitioners* are trained in arthritis and related illnesses and can assist your doctor with treatment. They also help teach you about your treatment program and can answer many of your questions or direct you to other resources for information.

Physician assistants are trained, certified and licensed to assist physicians by recording medical history and performing the physical examination, diagnosis and treatment of commonly encountered medical problems under the supervision of a licensed physician.

Physical therapists can show you exercises to help keep your muscles strong and your joints from becoming stiff. They can help you learn how to use special equipment to move better. Some physical therapists are trained to design individualized fitness programs for cardiovascular health maintenance and weight control. In general, physical therapists are concerned with larger joints – shoulders, hips and knees – and broad exercises, in contrast to *occupational therapists*, who are concerned with the hands and fine motor coordination.

Rehabilitation counselors can work with you to find solutions to work-related problems, such as job retraining or workplace modification.

Occupational therapists can teach you how to reduce strain on your joints while doing everyday activities. They can fit you with splints and other devices, if needed, to help reduce stress on your joints. Their role is mostly for problems with the small joints of the hands, and occasionally with arms and shoulders.

Pharmacists fill your prescriptions for medicines and can explain the actions and side effects of particular drugs. Pharmacists can tell you how different medicines work together and can answer questions about over-the-counter medications.

Social workers can help you access community resources, and they can help you find solutions to social and financial problems related to your arthritis. They may be of particular help in family situations such as helping to redistribute household responsibilities.

Getting the Most from Your Health-Care Team

Communication is the key to getting the most benefit from the health-care professionals on your team. The relationships you develop will probably be long-term ones, and will require work on both parts to develop trust and communication – much like a business partnership or a marriage. You should feel comfortable expressing your fears, asking questions you may think are "stupid" (but really aren't), and negotiating a treatment plan that all are satisfied with, without feeling that the health-care professionals are talking down to you or are not interested in your concerns.

There are two things to remember that will help to open (and keep open) the lines of communication. First, try to keep in mind that your doctor or therapist is only human. He or she gets tired, has headaches and even experiences bad days like you do. In addition, it's frustrating not to be able to cure someone with a chronic condition like arthritis. Health-care professionals must take their satisfaction from seeing improvements in your condition, such as an enhanced quality of life or fewer damaged joints, rather than cures.

Second, remember that the biggest threat to a good relationship and good communication is lack of time. When time is short, there may not be enough time to fully explain things or explore options. In medical offices today, the time your doctor has to be with you is very limited due to financial or insurance coverage reasons that may be beyond his or her control. Your health professionals' anxiety about time may lead to rushed messages that you misunderstand.

Make the most of your time with each health-care professional. Be prepared ahead of time with questions and any important changes in your condition that you wish to discuss. Remember – different health professionals can complement each other in some areas. More than one may be able to provide answers to some of your questions.

Taking P.A.R.T.

One way you can maximize the resources of your medical management team is by using a method called "Taking P.A.R.T." This technique involves preparing a list of

Take P.A.R.T.

To get the most out of your contacts with your medical management team, remember to take P.A.R.T.:

Prepare a list of questions, concerns and symptoms.

Ask questions.

Repeat what you have heard.

Take action to reduce barriers to treatments.

questions or concerns before your visit, asking questions, repeating what you heard and taking action by participating as fully as you can in treatment and management decisions.

Preparing involves making and keeping your appointment, keeping a diary or journal of your symptoms and your medications, and writing down the questions you want answered. Make a list of all your medications, including dosages, and keep it in your wallet for easy access. Be sure to include over-the-counter medications and supplements, too, as these substances can have interactions with prescription drugs your doctor gives you. It's all too easy to forget about important questions or exact dosages of drugs in the hustle and bustle of the doctor's office.

Asking your questions may take a little time, but your doctor understands these are valid concerns you have about your disease or your treatment. Bringing a prioritized list of questions to your appointment can save time and may bring up valuable information concerning your treatment.

Repeating the information or instructions you receive back to your health-care professional is a great way to make sure you have heard the information correctly and that you understand it. Taking notes may also help you remember complicated instructions. Feel free to ask for any available written handouts or instructions.

Taking action means you are personally involved in decisions about your treatment. This step is important because it allows you to share information about your goals and preferences. Let your doctor or other health-care professional know about your feelings, your lifestyle and your concerns. If something does not work, let him or her know so you can try something else.

Chapter 10

Medical Management:

Effective Strategies for Treatment

Good living with rheumatoid arthritis involves much more than drugs, but powerful new medications approved in the last decade have had the greatest impact on rheumatoid arthritis outlook in the history of the disease's treatment. Self-management, exercise and a positive outlook can make a big difference in how you feel on a day-to-day basis. Yet medications are the cornerstone of RA treatment for most people. Although there is no cure, excellent control of inflammation to reduce pain and functional limitations is now possible in most people with rheumatoid arthritis.

Doctors now have a much better understanding of the whole disease process than they did even ten or 20 years ago. This deeper understanding of the way rheumatoid arthritis works led to the evolution of new treatment strategies with more effective medications. In addition to the introduction of new drugs, doctors now utilize older drugs in new ways, and pinpoint drug combinations that may be more helpful than using one drug at a time. These developments make the outlook for people with rheumatoid arthritis much better than at any time since the disease was first described.

Acute vs. Chronic Disease

In Chapter 1, we discussed some of the differences between acute and chronic diseases. Acute diseases, such a pneumonia or influenza, have a specific cause (such as a bacterium or virus), and usually have a relatively defined duration – say, a week or a month.

In an acute illness, doctors usually follow a set protocol or treatment to cure the disease. The patient is often a passive participant. He or she is only required to follow the doctor's orders and take the medications prescribed. When a person has an acute infection, doctors, nurses and other health-care professionals make most of the decisions – including which drugs to take, when to take them and what other measures are necessary. A laboratory test identifies an appropriate antibiotic, the doctor prescribes it, and the pharmacist fills the prescription. Even if the acute disease is severe and life-threatening, the outcome is known within a week or two. Many acute diseases are self-limited, such as the common cold or even a mild musculoskeletal sports injury. Drugs may cure these, hasten the recovery process or simply make a person feel better. Soon, in most cases, the person is back to normal.

In chronic illness, it's a very different story. Treatment cannot be regarded as a cure, but rather as a means to control symptoms and prevent damage. Although recommendations regarding which drugs to take and when to take them are made by doctors, nurses and other health-care professionals, you – the patient – are the one who implements these decisions. You must make daily decisions that affect your well-being and your overall outcome: Whether or not to exercise, what to eat, whether or not to adapt your movements or use assistive devices, whether or not to take your medications as prescribed, whether or not to seek massage therapy or other complementary pain-relief techniques. The outcome of your chronic disease, unlike acute illness, may not be known for 10 to 20 years. If you have a chronic disease like RA, you have a great deal more control over your own management and outcome than a person with an acute illness. You become, in a sense, your own case manager.

One Drug vs. Many Drugs

Let's distinguish between diseases for which a single "best" drug can be identified and diseases in which there are many different "best" drugs. Again, many of our ideas about the treatment of diseases are derived from the treatment of an infectious disease. In an infectious disease, we sometimes forget that although a person may appear to be cured by taking an antibiotic, the target of the antibiotic is not the person, but rather a specific microorganism. In this setting, a drug that works in one person is likely to work equally well in other people with the same infection, taking into consideration that some people may have allergic reactions to certain drugs and may need an alternative treatment. It's usually possible to identify the "best" drug for a given infection, because the same microorganism is involved in each case.

In treating rheumatoid arthritis, people are complex and differ from one another in genetic makeup, levels of nutrition, age, lifestyle, background and many other factors that may affect the choice of drug. Therefore, there is no single best drug for all people, although there certainly is evidence that certain drugs are better in more people than other drugs. Naming the best drug for all people with rheumatoid arthritis is a little like trying to name the best flavor of ice cream for all people: The best selling flavor might be preferred by most people, but there will always be some people who like another flavor better.

The "Old" Approach to Medical Management

The medical approach to treating rheumatoid arthritis, as well as other chronic diseases, is based on a principle to "do no harm." That is, the treatment prescribed should not be worse than the disease itself. This remains a valid principle in any type of medical care – as long as the judgment of what is harmful is based on a realistic assessment of how harmful the disease might be.

In the old approach, sometimes called the pyramid approach, doctors were concerned that many of the drugs might be more harmful to people than the rheumatoid arthritis.

Doctors started at the base of the pyramid with first-line drugs, such as nonsteroidal anti-inflammatory drugs (NSAIDs) or salicylates (the most common of which is aspirin), along with simple measures such as patient education and physical therapy. If these medicines did not control the disease, doctors then moved up the pyramid to the more powerful disease-modifying antirheumatic drugs (DMARDs) and immunosuppressive drugs. Progressing up the pyramid could take quite a while, because the effectiveness of many of the drugs cannot be determined until after a considerable period of time – sometimes even several months.

The problem with applying this approach to rheumatoid arthritis was that, in the past, doctors did not have a complete understand-

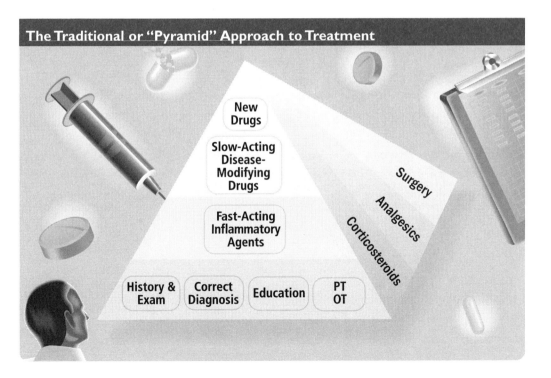

The Traditional or "Pyramid" Approach to Treatment

New Drugs

Slow-Acting Disease-Modifying Drugs

Surgery

Analgesics

Fast-Acting Inflammatory Agents

Corticosteroids

History & Exam   Correct Diagnosis   Education   PT OT

ing of the disease process or the amount of joint damage that could result in the first few years of this chronic condition. Research has shown that in the first two years of persistent arthritis, joint damage is likely to have already begun. Once these factors were understood, the strategy of treatment changed and doctors began prescribing more powerful medicines earlier in the course of the disease.

Another problem with the old approach to treatment is that some of the older drugs, such as gold injections and penicillamine, have a much higher likelihood of side effects than newer drugs, such as etanercept, infliximab, adalimumab, anakinra or methotrexate. The newer drugs have allowed more aggressive approaches to the management of rheumatoid arthritis at an earlier stage of the disease, when joint damage may still be prevented.

The New Approach: A Preventive Strategy

Now, doctors prescribe powerful drugs early in the disease course in an effort to control inflammation and prevent damage to joints. This new approach is similar to the early, aggressive treatment of high blood pressure to prevent long-term damage to the heart and blood vessels. There is no point in hiding the fact that rheumatoid arthritis can lead to severe long-term outcomes. By recognizing and even emphasizing the possible damage to the body that may result from a disease, doctors, other health professionals, patients, and their friends and families may be mobilized to act to prevent these consequences.

This approach to prevention has made a big difference in cardiovascular disease and is now making a big difference in rheumatoid arthritis. For most people with RA, rheumatologists use combinations of available drugs to find the right treatment program for each individual. In fact, most people must take at least two drugs to adequately control disease, and many people take three or four different drugs.

Is This New Approach Safe?

The old approach to treating rheumatoid arthritis was slow and often produced disappointing results. In addition, some of the drugs thought to be less harmful actually had fairly severe side effects and led to poor long-term outcomes. Many people with rheumatoid arthritis had lost hope. What about the new approach? Is it really more effective? And are these new drugs safe?

Evidence is still incomplete on the long-term effects of taking several drugs – especially the powerful, disease-modifying ones – in combination to treat rheumatoid arthritis. There is the possibility they could be more toxic than each drug taken alone. However, research studies indicate that combinations of drugs are no more likely to cause side effects than drugs taken individually. Aggressive therapy, including drug combinations, has the very real potential to minimize joint damage that previously occurred during the early years of disease in some people. And of course, as always, you must keep in mind that different people have different responses to these medications. Some individuals will do just fine with a conservative approach, but others will obviously need the more aggressive treatment strategies.

The issue is really not so much "Is my disease so bad that I need the aggressive treatment?" but rather, "Can I be better off in five years with aggressive treatment?" It is now known that the "side effects" of rheumatoid arthritis itself are considerably worse than the side effects of many of the new drugs used to treat the disease. Doctors have refined the dosages necessary to achieve good results with drugs, and keep side effects in mind as they prescribe medications to treat your disease.

Personally Speaking Stories from real people with rheumatoid arthritis

"**A**fter being diagnosed three years ago (following a diagnosis of Lyme disease the year before), I've had some good times and some bad ones. These past few months have been hard. I am an otherwise healthy, 47-year-old teacher, but the RA makes me really tired and dependent on others for certain tasks. I'm afraid that I may fall getting out of the bath, and rather crabby when it comes to doing things like the dishes, because it hurts! (Isn't that a great excuse for skipping the housework?!)

Learning to Adapt: Shortcuts and Screams
by Margaret Isham,
Cape Cod, MA

"I'm a very independent single mother with a wonderful boyfriend, and when he tries to help me out more than I like, I say, "No, I am fine," which drives him crazy because it is obvious that I am not! Therefore, I am learning to accept more help and not be so independent. That is very hard for me.

"I have been learning to adapt in many ways. I try different types of toothpaste as it is hard to squeeze it out of the tube. Once a pill bottle is open, I move the whole contents to a baggie, as the bottles are hard to open. I cut packages, bags of cat food and kitty litter open instead of trying to rip them.

"I have actually screamed at the RA once or twice when I am alone in the house and feeling frustrated. I feel a bit crazy, but it's good to let it out as I am a very mild-mannered, easy-going person who never screams! I have had to give up the treadmill and lifting weights, but when I can, I do Pilates and yoga. Next will be swimming. I am not someone who likes swimming very much and where I live, there is only one place to swim unless you like frigid ocean temperatures, so I am a little limited there.

"I sometimes worry about my future. I do not want to be a bed-ridden old hag, and there are sure days I feel like one. I certainly have needed to become quieter and more sedate. No more wild and crazy nights out!"

What You Can Do

You play a vital role in your own RA treatment. Learn about the drugs your doctor prescribes: how they work, the benefits and their potential side effects. Keep track of how your drugs seem to be working and what side effects you have, and share this information with your doctor during your appointments. Alert your doctor early to signs of a particular side effect so your medication can be reduced or changed as appropriate. Also, be sure to take your medication according to the doctor's instructions because this can help prevent or minimize side effects.

On the following three pages, you'll find worksheets to help you prepare for each doctor's visit, to talk openly with your doctor during the visit, and to better understand your medications and how to take them. Feel free to photocopy these worksheets and use them for each new doctor's visit.

Rheumatoid arthritis takes a different course in every person with the disease. So your specific needs and reactions to the drugs may differ from those of others. It is *your* needs and reactions that your doctor will consider first when developing or changing your treatment program.

Stopping Drug Treatment

Your medications may make you feel greatly improved. You may even be tempted, at certain points, to discontinue drug therapy because you feel so good. Stopping the therapy may be all right for a few weeks or even months. However, in most patients, a relapse is almost inevitable, usually within several weeks or months. In addition, getting the disease back under control will often be more difficult. It may be hard for you to continue to take drugs when there is no evidence of disease, but most experts recommend this approach. The best strategy is to keep things as normal as possible to prevent damage, which includes giving treatment when there is no evidence of the condition.

In the next chapter, we'll discuss the many drugs available to treat rheumatoid arthritis, including new medications that have changed the course of RA treatment entirely.

"ASK THE DOCTOR" Worksheet

Complete This Part Before Your Doctor's Visit

1. What is the main reason I am going to the doctor?

_____

_____

2. Is there anything else that concerns me about my health or treatment (e.g., effect of rheumatoid arthritis on work, family or mood; problems following the recommended treatment plan)?
_____Yes_____No

_____

3. What do I want the doctor to do today?

_____

_____

4. The symptoms that bother me the most are ... (What? Where? When did they start? Do they change over time? How long do they last?). NOTE: bring copies of any completed self-monitoring forms/diaries.

_____

_____

5. What medications (prescriptions and over-the-counter) am I taking regularly? (List name(s) and dosage or take the bottles to your appointment.)

_____

_____

6. What are my goals for treatment (what I want or expect to get out of treatment)?

_____

_____

7. Prepare and prioritize a list of questions to give the doctor early in the visit.

_____

_____

_____

8. Do I need Medicare, Medicaid or other insurance cards/forms today? _____Yes _____ No

_____

"ASK THE DOCTOR" Worksheet

Questions to ask your doctor during the visit.

1. What is happening to me? How is my rheumatoid arthritis likely to affect me?

_____

_____

2. What are the results of my tests and what do they mean? May I have a copy of the results?

_____

3. Why do I need the lab tests or X-rays that you are recommending today?

_____

4. Are there any risks from these tests?

_____

5. When should I call for the results?

_____

6. What should I do at home (diet, activity, treatment options, special instructions, medications, precautions, etc.)?

_____

_____

a. What are the benefits, costs and drawbacks (or risks) for each option for treatment?

_____

b. How and how often do I do the treatment? _____

_____

c. How long should I give it a try? _____

_____

7. When should I call if my condition doesn't get better and the treatment does not seem to be working? What additional symptoms would warrant my calling before my next scheduled visit?

_____

_____

8. When should I return for another visit?

_____

"ASK THE DOCTOR" Worksheet

Medication questions:

1. What is the name of the drug?_____

2. What are the purpose and benefits of this drug?

   _____

3. How quickly does it work? How long should I take this drug?

   _____

4. What are the possible side effects or drawbacks to the drug?

   _____

a. When should I contact you about side effects?

   _____

b. What can I do to prevent or deal with the side effects or drawbacks?

   _____

5. Is it all right to take the drug with other drugs (such as cold, sinus, allergy, pain medicines)
   I am taking? _____Yes _____No
   If not, what drugs should I avoid? _____

   _____

6. When is the best time to take the drug? Before, with or after meals? _____

7. What should I do if I forget to take my medicine?

   _____

8. Are there any changes I should make in my diet? _____Yes _____No
   If so, what?_____

a. Can I drink alcohol while taking this drug? _____Yes _____No

b. Are there any other restrictions? _____Yes _____No
   If so, what?_____

9. Should I avoid driving or any other activity while taking this drug? _____Yes _____No

10. Is a generic drug available? If so, is the generic form as effective? _____Yes _____No

Chapter 11

Aggressive Therapy:

Drugs to Treat Rheumatoid Arthritis

Good living with rheumatoid arthritis involves a great deal of self-management activities including diet, exercise and dealing positively with stress. But the most important component of treatment of rheumatoid arthritis is your drugs. A number of new, effective drugs have emerged in recent years to change the face of RA treatment entirely. In this chapter, we'll go over the many categories of drugs used to treat this disease, the specific medications used, and other important issues associated with your RA drugs.

You also play an important role in this area of your RA treatment. While only your doctor can prescribe many of the drugs included in this chapter, you must work hard to take them properly, regularly and according to your doctor's instructions. You must keep track of the other drugs you take – even for conditions other than your arthritis, such as high blood pressure, headaches or sleep problems, if you have them – and even herbs and supplements you try. You must check the prescriptions your pharmacist dispenses to make sure you are getting the correct medicine, and you must keep track of changes in your insurance coverage of drugs. Most importantly, you must stay well informed about the drugs for rheumatoid arthritis. This chapter will provide a good basis for your RA drug education. At the end of this book, you will find more resources, including how to contact the Arthritis Foundation chapter in your area, to get updated information about drug treatments.

Prescription vs.
Over-the-Counter Drugs

Drugs can be categorized in many ways, but the most basic distinction you must understand is this: Some drugs are available only by *prescription* and others are available *over the counter.* A prescription medication is one that you must have a doctor's written order – or phone call to the pharmacy – to receive and use legally. Over-the-counter or

OTC drugs can be purchased without a prescription, either at drugstores, supermarkets, convenience stores, or over the Internet. But OTC drugs are serious medications, too. Many OTC drugs come in stronger doses by prescription only.

Arthritis medications you'll find over the counter are the analgesic medication acetaminophen (*Tylenol*) and four nonsteroidal anti-inflammatory drugs (NSAIDs) – ibuprofen (*Advil, Motrin*), naproxen sodium (*Aleve*), ketoprofen (*Orudis KT*) and aspirin (*Bayer, Bufferin*). Although these drugs come in many formulations and in combinations with other ingredients (such as caffeine to speed pain relief, antihistamines to cause drowsiness, or a diuretic to ease menstrual bloating) these are the only over-the-counter medications you'll find to ease pain. These drugs often come in generic "store brands" as well, carrying the label of the store you purchased them in (such as pharmacy chains or supermarkets).

More and more, prescription drugs are becoming available over the counter, usually in lower doses. On the positive side, getting a medication has never been more convenient and less expensive. You don't need an appointment with a physician if all you need is something to ease the pain of an occasional headache or muscle strain. On the negative side, people are more likely than ever to medicate themselves with readily available drugs – not consulting their doctor. A 2004 report at the annual American Gastroenterological Association meeting suggested that many people take more OTC pain relievers than is necessary or safe, increasing the risk of serious stomach problems.

You may think that any drug you can buy over the counter is safe to use as you please, adjusting the dosage as you see fit. This is not true. It's important to follow the directions on the labeling exactly. You also should contact your doctor promptly if you suspect an adverse reaction or side effect to taking OTC drugs, or if symptoms don't improve.

OTC drugs may contain similar (or identical) active ingredients to the prescription drugs you take. So taking an over-the-counter medication such as *Advil* along with your prescription of *Motrin* may lead to an overdose. Tell your doctor about *all* the medications you are taking at any time, including over-the-counter medicines. Fortunately, most OTC medications have new labels that help you understand the active ingredients inside and how to take them properly. OTC medications that don't have the labels yet will be required by law to have them shortly.

In the coming sections, we'll look more closely at the general categories of drugs used to treat rheumatoid arthritis. Most of these drugs are available by a doctor's prescription only at this time. At the end of the chapter, we provide a handy drug chart that you can use to quickly look up important information about each of these drugs.

Nonsteroidal Anti-Inflammatory Drugs (NSAIDs)

Nonsteroidal anti-inflammatory drugs or NSAIDs are drugs similar to aspirin that can reduce inflammation. In reducing inflammation, these drugs also relieve pain. There are three generations of these drugs. The first generation is aspirin, which, in its non-coated form, is often quite irritating to the stomach when taken on a regular basis, as many people with chronic illness must do. The second generation is other forms of aspirin (such as enteric-coated and zero-order release aspirin) and drugs such as ibuprofen (*Motrin, Advil*), naproxen (*Naprosyn, Aleve*), indomethacin (*Indocin*) and others. These are often as effective as aspirin, but with less irritation to the stomach. Most recently, a third generation of NSAIDs known as COX-2 inhibitors, including celecoxib (*Celebrex*), rofecoxib (*Vioxx*) and valdecoxib (*Bextra*), has been developed. These drugs can offer greater safety from gastrointestinal problems.

NSAIDs reduce (and sometimes even eliminate) inflammation, and thereby lessen pain in people with rheumatoid arthritis. Joint inflammation results from the production of certain chemicals called *cytokines*, which, in turn, stimulate a subgroup of chemicals called prostaglandins. A primary action of NSAIDs is to inhibit production of prostaglandins, which in turn reduces the inflammation and pain associated with rheumatoid arthritis.

As we discussed in Chapter 2, inflammation normally serves to protect the body from invasion by an infection or bacterium, and to help heal wounds such as a cut or fracture. Therefore, when regulated properly, prostaglandins and cytokines are not in the body to be harmful, but to protect us. When inflammation has accomplished its mission, the production of its chemicals should "shut off" through complex control mechanisms. But in people with RA, inflammation does not shut off. Prostaglandins and cytokines are produced when they shouldn't be, leading to inflammation, pain and long-term damage.

NSAIDS AND STOMACH DISTRESS

In addition to their role in inflammation, prostaglandins are also normally found in certain tissues and organs to perform necessary functions. Prostaglandins help protect the lining of the stomach from acid, which can eat away at the stomach and cause bleeding or a hole in the stomach called an *ulcer*. Ulcers can be very serious. Because NSAIDs reduce the production of prostaglandins, they may cause stomach irritation and undesirable gastrointestinal side effects.

Prostaglandins also aid in removal of fluid from the kidneys, maintain a balance of competing chemicals in the brain, and promote normal blood clotting in platelets. That's why NSAIDs may cause problems with kidney function, such as fluid retention; central nervous system function, such as headaches and feeling "spacey"; or interfere with normal blood clotting. The possible bleeding problem is the reason surgeons ask patients to stop taking NSAIDs for a week or two prior to any surgery. Some of the newer NSAIDs cause fewer of these types of problems. We'll discuss those new treatments later in the section.

ASPIRIN: THE CLASSIC NSAID

Aspirin has been used as a medicine since ancient times. Long ago, people realized that eating the bark of the willow tree, or drinking a tea brewed from the bark, could help treat pain and certain illnesses. In the late 19th century, the active chemical in willow bark (called *salicylate*) was synthesized as a pill. Thus, modern aspirin was born.

Aspirin remains a very effective drug for relief of inflammation and pain. However, plain aspirin is too irritating to the stomach for long-term use in the high quantities needed for treating rheumatoid arthritis. Newer forms of aspirin including *Ascriptin* (aspirin mixed with *Maalox*), enteric-coated aspirin (*Ecotrin*) and zero-order release aspirin (*ZORprin*) were created. These drugs cause much lower levels of stomach irritation. Even when aspirin is not absorbed in the stomach (for instance, when it is given as a suppository through the rectum or as a zero-order release aspirin absorbed in the small intestine), some stomach irritation occurs, indicating that general systemic effects of aspirin lead to stomach irritation.

Nonetheless, research studies showed that the newer, less irritating forms of aspirin were favored by more people with rheumatoid arthritis than any of the other NSAIDs available before 1990. There is still a place for aspirin and its spin-offs in the treatment of certain people with rheumatoid arthritis.

OTHER TRADITIONAL NSAIDS

Beginning in the 1970s, a number of other NSAIDs were developed by the pharmaceutical industry and are now widely used. Indomethacin (*Indocin*) and ibuprofen (*Motrin, Advil, Nuprin*) were among the first developed. (Ibuprofen is available over the counter in lower doses.) These anti-inflammatory drugs did not have the same chemical composition as aspirin, and many people found them easier to take. Nonetheless, these NSAIDs carried with them the same potential side effects as aspirin – irritation of the stomach, interference with removal of fluid by the kidneys, imbalance in the central nervous system and reduced blood clotting – although at lower levels.

Indomethacin is usually not very helpful to most people with rheumatoid arthritis, although a few people experience great benefit. Indomethacin may cause unacceptable headaches and "spacey" feelings in more people than any other NSAID. But everyone is different – one of the recurring themes of this book – so if only two percent of people with rheumatoid arthritis may benefit substantially from indomethacin use, that drug is well worth trying for those few people.

Ibuprofen was the first major alternative to aspirin and was launched with great fanfare. Many people who take ibuprofen experience as much pain relief as with aspirin, but have less gastrointestinal discomfort. In addition, there is a lower risk of severe gastrointestinal irritation and events than with aspirin. Ibuprofen is the most widely used NSAID, particularly since 1992 when it became available over the counter as *Advil, Nuprin, Motrin* or *Mediprin*. However, the nonprescription

200-mg dose is often not sufficient for people with rheumatoid arthritis, although it may be quite effective for a relatively minor trauma such as a strained muscle. People with rheumatoid arthritis often need 400, 600 or even 800 mg of ibuprofen several times a day to gain effective pain relief.

One drawback to the use of ibuprofen, aspirin and other traditional NSAIDs is that they must be taken at least three or four times per day to give people the best benefit, because their effects only last for a few hours. This problem led scientists to develop longer-acting NSAIDs, which only need to be taken twice or even once per day. Some

of the more widely used long-acting NSAIDs include naproxen (*Naprosyn*), which is available in doses of 250, 375 and 500 mg, and also is available without a prescription as *Aleve* in a dose of 220 mg. Other twice-a-day compounds include nabumetone (*Relafen*), ketoprofen (*Orudis, Oruvail*) and diclofenac (*Voltaren*). Indomethacin also comes in a slow release form for twice daily usage (*Indocin SR*). Some of the once-a-day NSAIDs include piroxicam (*Feldene*) and oxaprozin (*Daypro*). Although these newer NSAIDs are taken less frequently, they still have the same potential gastrointestinal side effects of NSAIDs.

Personally Speaking Stories from real people with rheumatoid arthritis

"The symptoms began six years ago. In fact, RA seemed like it blew in the window one night because I was always healthy until then. I awoke with fingers that looked like sausages, so stiff that I couldn't bend them, hot to the touch and red, sore and swollen.

Positive Attitude: Stay on Top of RA and Beat It!
by Linda Knittle, Decatur, IN

"Diagnosis: RA. I was devastated when the doctor told me, and being a nurse, I knew it was serious. I was sent to a rheumatologist, and treatment began immediately. I didn't adjust to having this dreadful disease very well. Depression set in. For the first time in my life, I could not do the everyday things we take for granted.

"I'm now doing my best to stay active. I can't walk due to my bad feet and ankles, so I go to a pool three times a week and water walk. This way, I'm moving all my muscles and it doesn't hurt. I try to stay positive, because I will not let this disease get the best of me. I will stay on top of it and beat it!

"I pray there will soon be a cure for this disease. Something more needs to be done for people that have arthritis, due to its disabling tendencies and the high cost of the medication. I will not give up. I will fight with all my might and I will hope and pray for a cure."

THE GASTROINTESTINAL DILEMMA

The problem of gastrointestinal irritation was recognized in the 1980s as a major problem in the use of NSAIDs in all forms of arthritis. Several types of research studies indicated that every year about one of every 50 to 100 people who took an NSAID regularly would experience a major gastrointestinal event, such as bleeding ulcer or perforation, leading to hospitalization. One in 50 to 100 people may not sound like a lot of people, but if millions of people take these drugs, then thousands of people could expect to have serious side effects from the use of NSAIDs.

One important NSAID-related gastrointestinal side effect is that a person might experience an acute problem such as internal bleeding, a hole or perforation, or an obstruction in the stomach without any warning signs or symptoms such as pain, nausea or heartburn. By contrast, other people may have many symptoms and never experience a serious gastrointestinal event. Therefore, although patients and doctors respond primarily to symptoms – that is, reports of heartburn or stomach pain – the major reason to be concerned about the gastrointestinal tract may not be pain, but risk of a serious event. This risk increases substantially in people over age 75, those with a previous history of gastrointestinal events and those with more active, severe joint disease.

The risk of serious stomach effects prevents many people from taking traditional NSAIDs. With earlier use of disease-modifying antirheumatic drugs (DMARDs), as we discussed in Chapter 10, NSAIDs are no longer regarded as the mainstay of the treatment of rheumatoid arthritis. Yet more than 60 percent of RA patients continue to take these drugs, more for their ability to relieve pain than for their anti-inflammatory activity. NSAIDs are widely used for treating other rheumatic conditions, including osteoarthritis, tendinitis and bursitis. Because they are useful, widely used drugs, here are four strategies to help reduce gastrointestinal side effects of NSAIDs:

• **Combine NSAIDs with antacid drugs.** The first strategy involves the addition of drugs that might protect the lining of the stomach. One of the early attempts was a combination of aspirin and *Maalox* (*Ascriptin*), which many people found to cause less gastrointestinal irritation than plain aspirin. However, there was still a substantial rate of gastrointestinal ulcers and irritation – apparently due the fact that aspirin's chemical properties still irritated the stomach. Therefore, this strategy helped alleviate some symptoms, but it did not necessarily reduce the risk of serious events.

• **Add H2 blockers.** During the 1970s, a new class of compounds was developed called H2 blockers. These agents included cimetidine (*Tagamet*), famotidine (*Pepcid*), ranitidine (*Zantac*) and nizatidine (*Axid*). Now, many of these drugs are available over the counter as well as in prescription form. H2 blockers act by blocking receptors in the stomach that lead to the production of acid. The net result is less acid production. There is some reduction of the gastrointestinal irritation associated with NSAIDs with these drugs, but the protection provided by H2 blockers is far from complete.

• **Combine with synthetic prostaglandins.** Researchers have developed a pill that contains a synthetic prostaglandin called misoprostol (*Cytotec*). When taken with an NSAID, it helps to protect the stomach locally from irritation. Another drug that contains diclofenac (*Voltaren*) coated with misoprostol (*Arthrotec*) is another option. *Arthrotec* can be taken twice per day, and many people have found this a very effective drug.

• **Add proton pump inhibitors.** More recently, a class of gastrointestinal compounds known as *proton pump inhibitors* has become available that often provides even more effective relief than H2 blockers. Examples include omeprazole (*Prilosec*) (also now available in an over-the-counter dosage), lansoprazole (*Prevacid*) and esomaprazole magnesium (*Nexium*). Studies have documented that proton pump inhibitors can protect the stomach against the gastrointestinal side effects associated with NSAIDs because they block the secretion of acid into the stomach more effectively than H2 blockers.

COX-2 SPECIFIC INHIBITORS

During the 1990s, it was discovered that two types of enzymes called cyclooxygenase enzymes, or COX enzymes, lead to the synthesis of prostaglandins. Cyclooxygenase-1 (COX-1) is associated with many of the "healthy" functions of prostaglandins, such as protecting the lining of the stomach, helping to remove fluids, maintaining balance in the central nervous system and promoting blood clotting. Cyclooxygenase-2 (COX-2) is associated with some other functions of prostaglandins, including the inflammatory response.

In theory, a drug that inhibits COX-2 but not COX-1 would be able to inhibit the inflammatory response that occurs in rheumatoid arthritis without having the undesirable effects of some of the traditional NSAIDs, particularly the possibility of irritating the stomach and causing gastrointestinal events such as bleeding and perforation of the stomach. But there is some new concern that COX-2 drugs, because they do not inhibit COX-1 as well, may not provide the protection against cardiovascular problems (heart attacks and strokes) that regular NSAIDs (such as low-dose aspirin, a common preventive treatment for cardiovascular disease) provide. In addition, it may take years of study before doctors know how safe COX-2 drugs really are in preventing serious gastrointestinal complications.

Three selective COX-2 inhibitors are currently available on the market: celecoxib (*Celebrex*), rofecoxib (*Vioxx*) and valdecoxib (*Bextra*). A new COX-2 drug, etoricoxib (*Arcoxia*), is being considered by the FDA for approval.

DO NSAIDS HAVE A ROLE IN THE FUTURE OF RA TREATMENT?

The role of NSAIDs in rheumatoid arthritis is being reassessed. Previously it was suggested that NSAIDs should be used in all RA patients as the first line of therapy. However, with the availability of powerful new disease-modifying antirheumatic drugs (DMARDs), NSAIDs may not be needed in some people.

Many doctors are now using NSAIDs primarily for their analgesic (pain-relieving) properties. These drugs are able to relieve pain over and above their capacity to relieve inflammation. Very few people with rheumatoid arthritis are treated with NSAIDs alone now, because of evidence that NSAIDs alone are not sufficient to block the progression of joint destruction and functional disability. Instead, they may be used in combination with DMARDs to achieve the best possible control of pain and inflammation.

Analgesics

Analgesic drugs specifically relieve pain without necessarily having an effect on inflammation. The prototype drug in this class is acetaminophen (*Tylenol*), which may be combined with other pain-relieving drugs such as codeine. Acetaminophen is the drug that the American College of Rheumatology recommends as the first response to general arthritis pain. Another widely used analgesic drug is propoxyphene (*Darvon*). In addition, there are stronger narcotic analgesic drugs such as meperidine (*Demerol*), morphine, and compounds such as *Percocet*, *Percodan*, *Vicodin*, and others.

Analgesic drugs relieve pain because they act on the brain or the central nervous sys-

tem, which is where pain is perceived. As discussed in Chapter 2, it is generally better for rheumatoid arthritis pain to be relieved by controlling inflammation through the use of anti-inflammatory drugs. However, in certain patients at certain times – and in people who have painful joints as a result of joint damage, but no longer have active inflammation – it is often helpful to use analgesic drugs specifically to relieve pain. In addition, you may need analgesics to relieve other painful problems, such as a tooth extraction or menstrual cramps.

PAIN: IT'S ALL IN YOUR HEAD

Sometimes people confronted with severe pain may ask, "Is all of this pain in my head?" Well, the correct answer is yes, sort of. All pain *is* experienced in the head, although it may reflect problems in an arm or leg. Inflammation in the joints of your hands may send signals that something is wrong through your central nervous system to your brain, which interprets the signals and responds with pain. If you have a fractured leg that needs to be manipulated, you may be given anesthesia and put to sleep, at which point there is no more pain. This is an important principle because it reminds us that the perception of pain can be greater or lesser depending, in part, on how it is interpreted in the brain.

Of course, sometimes pain cannot be explained by inflammation or structural changes. This common form of musculoskeletal pain is experienced by people who have fibromyalgia. People with rheumatoid arthritis may also have fibromyalgia, as discussed in Chapter 5, and may require additional therapy to treat these problems.

ACETAMINOPHEN (*TYLENOL*)

The most widely used analgesic drug in the United States is acetaminophen (*Tylenol*), which is also known as paracetamol (*Panadol*) in Europe. It is available over the counter in lower doses and under various brand names. Acetaminophen may be a good substitute for NSAIDs in some people when it comes to reducing fever or relieving pain. However, it is not a good substitute with respect to the reduction of inflammation, which is one of the primary actions of aspirin. There is a slight reduction of inflammation associated with the use of acetaminophen, but it is very minimal compared with aspirin. So although you can substitute acetaminophen for an aspirin when you have a headache or a toothache, you cannot substitute acetaminophen for aspirin for the inflammation in rheumatoid arthritis. At the least, it will not have the same potential value as an anti-inflammatory drug.

Acetaminophen is now recommended as the first drug to be used for osteoarthritis, which in effect is what a person with rheumatoid arthritis who has damaged joints may be experiencing. Therefore, acetaminophen may be helpful when pain is not the result of inflammation in a person who might have damage to joints from long-standing rheumatoid arthritis.

Acetaminophen is often combined with a narcotic. Most frequently it is mixed with codeine as *Tylenol #1, 2, 3* or *4*, containing 15, 30, 45 and 60 mg of codeine, respectively. This combination is used by doctors for conditions that may cause pain beyond the rheumatoid arthritis or to "tide you over" during a flare of disease activity. Acetaminophen as a single drug or as a compound is usually *not* an effective long-term drug to be used for treating rheumatoid arthritis.

NARCOTIC ANALGESICS

A number of narcotic analgesic drugs are used as pain relievers for people with rheumatoid arthritis. In general, these drugs relieve pain more effectively than anti-inflammatory drugs or non-narcotic analgesic drugs. They include codeine, meperidine (*Demerol*), propoxyphene (*Darvon*), morphine, oxycodone, hydrocodone and a newer drug, tramadol (*Ultram*), which can also be mixed with acetaminophen (*Ultracet*). These drugs are often used in combination with acetaminophen and other drugs.

A general rule of thumb in treating rheumatoid arthritis or other rheumatic diseases has been to avoid the use of narcotic drugs under any conditions. Although it is true that one should think twice about the use of narcotic drugs, this position has been slowly modified just as the position about prednisone and other drugs has been modified. It is now believed that many people may benefit from the judicious use of narcotic drugs. Although there is a certain danger of dependence, studies have shown that people who experience severe pain are unlikely to become addicted – in contrast to people who have no pain and take narcotic drugs for other types of effects on the brain, or for pleasure.

Different doctors have very different views of the use of narcotic drugs. In general, research studies show that doctors tend to underestimate pain experienced by their patients. This leads to "undermedication" on the part of the doctor and frustration on the part of the patient. The use of questionnaires with pain scores has been very helpful in documenting the severity of pain from a patient's perspective, and many doctors use these measures in routine care to judge the need for additional pain relief. Pain manage-

ment is now one of the fastest growing segments of medical treatment, and new emphasis is being placed on understanding pain management in medical schools. In some cities, special pain centers and pain clinics treat pain specifically, with most of their patients experiencing chronic pain.

A number of narcotic compounds are now available to treat pain. These drugs may be best used to treat painful flares or other events that might occur – most likely from a fracture or other severe acute event. These drugs include *Percodan*, *Percocet* and *Lortab*. Furthermore, narcotic compounds can be given in the form of a patch worn on the skin, such as the *Duragesic* patch. This may be helpful in certain situations: such as

The Narcotics Debate

Some doctors would never prescribe narcotics for RA pain, while others argue that they can be appropriate treatments for pain. If pain relief is not achieved with NSAIDs, COX-2 drugs, or other treatments, then narcotics may be considered for some people.

The decision to go this route requires patient counseling on dependency and expected side effects of narcotic drugs. Some physicians will require their patients to sign a contract that outlines appropriate use of the drugs and the physician's expectations regarding ongoing use. Here are what many doctors view as central issues in the debate:

Advantages:

- Narcotics are the most effective available medications for managing chronic pain.
- The majority of patients don't need narcotics. But those that do should have the option for a trial period.
- The addiction rate from narcotics is one percent. Addiction (compulsive, self-destructive use) is not the same as dependence (withdrawal symptoms if the drug is stopped abruptly).
- Less pain results in better functioning.

when a person experiences a compression fracture of the spine, which can be acutely painful but that heals over a few weeks to months without long-term consequences.

One simple analgesic drug that has been used extensively is propoxyphene (*Darvon*). This drug's effectiveness in relieving pain has been shown to be comparable to acetaminophen in the population. However, as with all drugs, some people find propoxyphene more effective than acetaminophen, just as other people may find acetaminophen more effective than propoxyphene.

Corticosteroids

Corticosteroids are naturally occurring compounds required by the body for carrying out normal life processes. When cortisone was first given to people with rheumatoid arthritis in 1948, it was thought to be a miracle drug and perhaps even the cure for the disease. Unfortunately, cortisone or prednisone – the most commonly used chemical form of cortisone – caused many serious side effects that often became worse than the disease itself.

From the 1950s through the 1980s, doctors recommended that cortisone or prednisone not be used at all in rheumatoid arthritis, except for treating the most severe complications. However, over the last 15 years it has been recognized that low doses of cortisone, such as 5 mg of prednisone or less, can be taken reasonably safely over long peri-

Disadvantages:

- When you use narcotics, you are treating pain solely as a symptom, without necessarily eliminating the factors that cause it. Therefore, narcotics should be used only in the context of a thorough medical management program.
- Dependence is an expected result of treatment.
- Narcotics will dull pain, but not eliminate it. In other words, they are not a "cure" for your arthritis.
- Tolerance to narcotics occurs after a time – from months to years – so that increasing the dosage is necessary to maintain the same level of response.
- Narcotics have side effects such as mental fuzziness, constipation, nausea, drowsiness and itching that only add to the side effects from your other medications.

If you feel that your pain is not sufficiently managed by the drugs you are currently taking, talk to your doctor about other options. For more information, read *The Arthritis Foundation's Guide to Pain Management*, available by calling (800) 283-7800 or at www.arthritis.org.

ods to prevent joint damage without introducing major side effects. Another common term for corticosteroids is *glucocorticoids*.

Probably no drugs used in the treatment of rheumatoid arthritis, or even in clinical medicine in general, evoke more controversy than this class. Corticosteroids are a group of hormones that are produced naturally by the *adrenal gland*, an internal organ situated above the kidney. These hormones help support the circulatory system and regulate body functions. All of us make about 25 mg to 35 mg of cortisol (our naturally occurring corticosteroid) each day to support vital body functions. All humans need a certain level of corticosteroids to sustain life itself.

One of the most important drugs in the treatment of rheumatoid arthritis is prednisone, a synthetically produced version of cortisone. Synthetically produced cortisone is roughly similar to cortisol in its activity as a corticosteroid. On the other hand, prednisone is about five times more powerful than cortisone – which means that 25–35 mg of cortisone are roughly equivalent to 5–7 mg of prednisone. Prednisone also comes in an injectable form called *Depo-Medrol* and *Solu-Medrol*. The most powerful corticosteroid is dexamethasone, which is about 10 times more powerful than cortisone, so that 25 mg of cortisone is equivalent to 2.5 mg of dexamethasone.

A number of serious side effects may occur when people take high doses of glucocorticoids over long periods. These include weight gain, "moon face" appearance, increased susceptibility to infection, diabetes, high blood pressure, cataracts, avascular necrosis of the hip and other bones, and osteoporosis (thinning of bones). There is also a naturally occurring condition called Cushing's syndrome or hyperadrenocorticism, in which too much cortisol is made due to a dysregulation in the adrenal gland or due to a hormone-producing tumor. People with this condition may develop the same serious symptoms as people who take high doses of corticosteroids over long periods.

HIGH-DOSE VS. LOW-DOSE CORTICOSTEROIDS

One of the functions of corticosteroids is to shut down the inflammatory response after it is no longer needed to protect the body from infections or other events that may "jump start" the immune system (see Chapter 2).

Your doctor may prescribe corticosteroids to treat a variety of inflammatory conditions ranging from an acute insect bite or poison ivy to serious rheumatic diseases like rheumatoid arthritis or systemic lupus. For certain conditions, such as an attack of asthma, high doses such as 20–60 mg of prednisone are given, often in a "*dose-pack.*" In this form, the amount of the drug is tapered down over the course of a week to treat subacute inflammatory conditions. Of course, people generally recover from these conditions, but the corticosteroids may hasten the recovery, make recovery more likely, or even be life-saving. Regardless, the action of the drugs is needed over only a few days.

In a chronic condition such as rheumatoid arthritis, higher doses of corticosteroids are used over longer periods of time, and the situation becomes more complex. One reason is that the inflammation stimulus continues rather than disappears. If the corticosteroid dose is tapered rapidly, as in a dose-pack, symptoms tend to return when the dose reaches a low level or the drug is discontinued. There may even be a strong "rebound" effect in which symptoms actually increase. Occasionally, some physicians use high doses of pills or an injection of corticosteroids that are then rapidly tapered to normal levels to control acute flares. But over long periods, an effort is made to maintain dosage at less than 5 mg of prednisone per day.

Most people with rheumatoid arthritis appear to respond to low doses of corticosteroid (such as 5 mg of prednisone or less) similar to those made naturally in the adrenal gland. The side effects of long-term, low-dose corticosteroid use are much less serious than those seen with high doses. Side effects may still be seen – thinning of the skin, easy bruising and poorer wound healing, for example – but most of the major consequences, such as diabetes, hypertension and weight gain, are only slightly or no more common than in the general population of people with chronic diseases.

Many rheumatoid arthritis specialists suggest that the capacity of low-dose corticosteroids to help people function from day to day, relieve pain and slow long-term joint damage makes their use worthwhile.

HISTORY OF USE OF CORTICOSTEROIDS IN RHEUMATOID ARTHRITIS

Cortisone was first produced in the laboratory in 1948. It was immediately apparent that cortisone could lead to major benefit in people with rheumatoid arthritis and other inflammatory conditions. The effects of cortisone appeared almost as a "miracle" in the improvement seen overnight in many people. Magazine articles in the popular press at the time described the dramatic effects of cortisone, and many believed there was finally a cure for rheumatoid arthritis.

This period of great hope lasted only a few years. By the early 1950s, it was recognized that high doses of corticosteroids over periods longer than a few weeks or months were associated with severe side effects. The consequences often appeared to be as bad as, or even worse than, the disease itself. The medical community concluded that it would be undesirable to use *any* corticosteroids to treat rheumatoid arthritis. From the 1960s to the 1980s, medical texts recommended that these drugs be used only as a last resort if a person could not function at all or developed a severe consequence such as vasculitis.

The medical community redefined its attitude on corticosteroids in the 1980s, when it was recognized that low doses of these drugs could be used over long periods with fewer side effects than those seen with high doses. The idea was not to use high-dose corticosteroids at all, but to prescribe them in low doses over long, even indefinite, periods. It was found that people could safely take prednisone in doses of 3 to 7.5 mg per day or less, which would yield most of the benefits of high doses with very few of the side effects. In 1992, it was found that 75 percent of people with rheumatoid arthritis under the care of rheumatologists in the United States were taking corticosteroids, mostly over long periods and in low doses.

Of course everyone is different. A few people experience psychological distress when they take *any* dose of corticosteroids beyond what is naturally made in the body. These people can't take prednisone at all. However, benefits can be seen in doses as low as 1 mg per day.

DISCONTINUING CORTICOSTEOIDS – SOME PRECAUTIONS

Long-term use of corticosteroids in rheumatoid arthritis signals the body's adrenal glands to stop manufacturing cortisol. Therefore, if someone experiences an unusual stress, such as an accident, major illness or surgery, the body can't produce the boost of corticosteroids that it needs. It becomes necessary to give extra amounts of the drug. Likewise, a person who has taken high doses for more than a few weeks cannot abruptly stop taking them. A person may experience confusion and even collapse from not having enough corticosteroids if they are stopped suddenly. So you must taper the

dose gradually while the adrenal glands, which make corticosteroids in the body, build up their capacity to produce normal amounts of cortisol. This process generally takes about a month or two.

CORTICOSTEROIDS BY INJECTION

In addition to different types of corticosteroid pills, these drugs may be given by injection in several ways. Four are discussed briefly here.

• **A simple intramuscular injection.** A simple injection in a muscle known as an *intramuscular injection* of a corticosteroid may be given to quiet a generalized flare of rheumatoid arthritis. Two compounds often used for these injections are triamcinolone (*Kenalog*) and methylprednisolone (*Depo-Medrol*). Some people may be treated with intramuscular injections every two months rather than taking oral corticosteroids. This type of injection often results in substantial benefit, which usually lasts from one to eight weeks. Any doctor or trained nurse can give an intramuscular injection.

• **Injection into a joint.** If a single joint is swollen out of proportion to other joints, it may be beneficial for a doctor to inject that joint directly with corticosteroid, usually after removing as much fluid as possible (a process called *aspiration*). Joints commonly injected include the knees, ankles, shoulders, elbows, wrists and knuckles. This type of injection may be very effective to quiet inflammation in a specific joint. The injection delivers a much higher concentration of the drug directly into the joint, and does not expose you to the potential side effects of generalized corticosteroids. Administration of an injection into a joint requires special training or experience.

• **Injection of corticosteroids in soft tissues.** Injections may be helpful for conditions such as tendinitis or bursitis (see Chapter 5) in which the site of inflammation involves the soft tissue near a joint, rather than the joint directly. For example, the drugs may be injected in the tissue around the wrist in people who have carpal tunnel syndrome, a condition in which there may be numbness and tingling in the fingers. A local corticosteroid injection may also be given at the base of a finger to relieve a "trigger finger," in which a finger does not open up normally, but suddenly with a trigger action. Corticosteroid may be injected into tender points in people who have fibromyalgia along with rheumatoid arthritis (see Chapter 5).

• **Intravenous injection.** Intravenous corticosteroid injections, sometimes in very high doses, are known as "pulses" (or "pulse therapy"). These pulses may be given in doses up to 1,000 mg, sometimes on three consecutive days. This treatment is effective but results are temporary, and many doctors think that low-dose, long-term corticosteroids are just as helpful to people with rheumatoid arthritis. Since the introduction of many other effective treatments, the use of corticosteroid pulses has declined considerably. However, this treatment may still be effective in certain situations.

CORTICOSTEROIDS AS THE ONLY DRUG TREATMENT

Corticosteroids may leave you feeling so well that it may seem you don't need further medication. However, it is unusual that these drugs can be effective as the *only* treatment for most people with rheumatoid arthritis. In general, an additional drug, usually a disease-modifying antirheumatic drug (DMARD) – such as methotrexate, sulfasalazine, hydroxychloroquine or others – is needed.

WHAT SHOULD YOU WORRY ABOUT WHEN TAKING PREDNISONE?

The side effects listed for prednisone mostly are associated with high doses of this drug, and include higher likelihood of a "moon face," weight gain, increased likelihood of developing hypertension, diabetes, osteoporosis and related fractures, and susceptibility to infections. Although these are not unusual in people who have taken *high* doses of prednisone, they are quite unusual in most people who have taken low doses, even over long periods. Many people have taken low-dose prednisone for more than 10 years and have normal bone densities. We must also remember that there is an increased likelihood of infection and osteoporosis associated with rheumatoid arthritis itself, which may be attributed to the corticosteroid treatment but may be simply a manifestation of the disease.

Disease-Modifying Antirheumatic Drugs (DMARDs)

Disease-modifying antirheumatic drugs, or DMARDs, are a subclass of drugs that modify the underlying mechanisms in the body that may be causing your rheumatoid arthritis symptoms. Many of these drugs were first used to treat entirely different diseases, but doctors found that they also had effects that might be useful in treating arthritis.

One of the most widely used and important DMARDs for treating rheumatoid arthritis is methotrexate (*Rheumatrex, Trexall*). Disease-modifying antirheumatic drugs appear to have the capacity to slow joint destruction in rheumatoid arthritis over time. Disease-modifying antirheumatic drugs are used in addition to nonsteroidal anti-inflammatory drugs and often prednisone.

One of the earliest DMARDs was injectable gold, which is still used effectively to treat some people. Other DMARDs include leflunomide (*Arava*), azathioprine (*Imuran*), chloroquine, hydroxychloroquine (*Plaquenil*), sulfasalazine (*Azulfidine*), and oral gold (*Ridaura*). Another drug is currently used to treat rheumatoid arthritis, although It's not technically a DMARD, but an antibiotic: minocycline (*Minocin*). It's often included in this category when discussing rheumatoid arthritis treatment.

Methotrexate

Methotrexate was first used in the 1940s to treat various forms of cancer, including leukemia and breast cancer, and was one of the first successful chemotherapy drugs. The main action of methotrexate in cancer is to kill cells that grow and divide without normal control mechanisms.

Rheumatoid arthritis is not a cancer, but in RA, cells in the joint don't act normally. Therefore, the idea of killing abnormally dividing cells makes sense. But there's a major difference in the strategy of killing cancer cells compared to killing cells in arthritis. If 99 percent of the cancerous cells are killed, the 1 percent that survive usually will continue to divide and cause disease to return to its previous level. But in rheumatoid arthritis, if 80 percent of abnormal cells are killed, the patient usually improves greatly. So much lower amounts of methotrexate are needed to treat RA – often less than one tenth as much as is used to treat cancer.

Although the original reason for using methotrexate to treat rheumatoid arthritis involved killing abnormal cells, it now seems likely that methotrexate works in rheumatoid arthritis primarily to fight inflammation.

HIGH-DOSE AND LOW-DOSE METHOTREXATE

A simple example can help illustrate the difference between a small dose and a large dose of methotrexate: It's like the difference between, say, a glass compared to a bottle of red wine. All bottles of wine have a warning that drinking the contents may be harmful to health, despite extensive evidence that one or two glasses a day of red wine are associated with living longer. However, one or two *bottles* a day of red wine are not associated with living longer, and in fact will probably shorten your life! Similarly, small doses of methotrexate may be quite safe and very beneficial, while large doses are appropriate only for certain situations in people with cancer.

High doses of methotrexate can come with many, severe side effects, including hair loss, mouth sores, decreased liver function and changes in blood counts. These side effects can be dangerous and could leave a person more vulnerable to infection. Low doses, however, infrequently cause changes in blood counts and liver function, although some hair loss can occur in some cases. Overall, low-dose methotrexate appears less likely to cause side effects than most drugs used in the treatment of rheumatoid arthritis, including many NSAIDs.

ARE YOU A CANDIDATE FOR METHOTREXATE?

When methotrexate was first used to treat rheumatoid arthritis, it was reserved for people whose cases were severe and long-lasting. Doctors were concerned that its side effects would not justify its use in people who had relatively mild cases of the disease. As might be expected, many of the first people to receive methotrexate as an RA treatment already had considerable joint damage. There was substantial improvement in these people, but most of them still experienced problems in functional disability and pain as their joints were irreparably damaged.

Over a nearly 25-year period of using methotrexate as a widespread treatment for RA, doctors now realize that low doses of the drug can control inflammation and prevent damage to joints. In addition, some of the newer RA treatments, such as leflunomide (*Arava*), etanercept (*Enbrel*), infliximab (*Remicade*), anakinra (*Kineret*) and adalimumab (*Humira*), which we'll discuss later in this chapter, may be as effective as methotrexate, perhaps even more effective. Over the next few years, more information will emerge about the long-term effectiveness of these new drugs, and this knowledge may reshape the face of RA treatment dramatically. In addition, there may be even newer drugs on the horizon that will have an even greater impact.

As with all drugs, some people cannot take methotrexate. Nonetheless, with evidence of few, manageable side effects, methotrexate is one of the most common treatments for rheumatoid arthritis. Many doctors believe all people who have rheumatoid arthritis should take some dose of methotrexate if they can tolerate it. The most feared consequences of methotrexate – liver damage and impaired production of blood cells – are quite unusual when it's used in low doses.

WHEN SHOULD YOU BEGIN METHOTREXATE?

Here again, recommendations are changing. Traditionally, methotrexate was saved for later in the disease course. Now, with a goal of preventing damage, the drug is used early to treat inflammation as aggressively as possible. Of course, certain people may be candidates for other treatments, such as biologic response modifiers (discussed on p. 95). In addition, newer, better, and possibly safer drugs may be on the approval horizon (see p. 104).

WHEN SHOULD METHOTREXATE BE DISCONTINUED?

Although all people prefer to discontinue drug treatment if possible, considerable evidence suggests that people who respond well to methotrexate and tolerate it should continue to take some dose on an indefinite basis. It's difficult to say you will use any drug forever, because it's possible that new and better treatments will be developed, or that the arthritis may remit. Medical research may some day find a drug or treatment that people with RA need to take for only a few weeks or months rather than indefinitely. However, until such treatments become available, long-term methotrexate treatment is one of the best ways for most people to control the inflammation of rheumatoid arthritis and prevent joint damage over many years.

WHEN SHOULD OTHER DRUGS BE ADDED?

Another shifting area of RA treatment is the combination of drugs. In the past, if you took a DMARD such as gold injections or penicillamine that seemed to work for a while and then seemed to stop working later, the doctor would discontinue that drug and begin another DMARD. Doctors felt that severe side effects were more likely if two powerful drugs were used together.

Methotrexate has far fewer side effects than most of the other drugs used to treat rheumatoid arthritis, so many doctors now add a second DMARD or biologic response modifier if methotrexate does not control swelling and pain entirely. "Combination therapy" with methotrexate and drugs such as hydroxychloroquine (*Plaquenil*), sulfasalazine (*Azulfidine*), etanercept (*Enbrel*), leflunomide (*Arava*), infliximab (*Remicade*) and others is now quite common.

Combining drugs to treat RA is similar to the way doctors manage other chronic conditions such as high blood pressure. If one drug gives partial control, they usually add a second drug rather than switching entirely from one drug to another. Sometimes a third, fourth and or even fifth drug may be added. Similarly, complete control of inflammation in rheumatoid arthritis may be achieved by using as many drugs as might be necessary and safe.

WHAT SHOULD YOU WORRY ABOUT WHEN TAKING METHOTREXATE?

A number of warnings are often given to patients concerning the use of methotrexate, which can often seem very distressing. Become familiar with the possible side effects of methotrexate and recognize that most of these are quite unusual.

• **Methotrexate can reduce the formation of normal blood cells.** A check of blood cell counts is needed every four to eight weeks. However, with low-dose methotrexate, decreases in blood counts are quite unusual, particularly when folic acid (readily available over the counter) is used as a supplement.

• **Methotrexate is a liver toxin.** Some doctors will suggest that you completely abstain from alcohol, although other doctors think one or two alcoholic drinks per day is reasonable. All doctors agree that heavy use of alcohol is very dangerous if you're taking methotrexate. Follow your doctor's advice. Patients using methotrexate should be given liver blood tests every four to six weeks to monitor the effect of the drug on the liver.

• **Methotrexate can cause a form of pneumonia.** We usually associate pneumonia with bacteria or some other type of infection, rather than with a chemical or drug. So this possible, serious effect of methotrexate is important to note. However, after the pneumonia is better, most people can take methotrexate again a few weeks later without any problem. Some doctors believe that there may be an infection, as well as methotrexate, causing the pneumonia. Nonetheless, the pneumonia gets better when you stop taking methotrexate.

• **Methotrexate can cause changes in the genetic structure of cells.** Such genetic structural change in cells theoretically makes a person vulnerable to development of cancer. However, this is very unlikely when low-dose methotrexate is used for RA treatment.

Many studies have shown that any possible increased risk of cancer in methotrexate-treated patients is minimal.

• **Methotrexate is teratogenic.** Teratogenic means that the drug can lead to a risk of abnormal development of a baby if a woman becomes pregnant while taking methotrexate. Therefore, women of child-bearing years who are not using birth control should not use methotrexate. Also, men should not take this drug if the couple is trying to conceive.

• **Methotrexate can cause hair loss.** Hair loss can often be controlled by reducing the dose of methotrexate. Sometimes discontinuation of the drug is necessary.

• **Methotrexate can cause mouth sores.** Mouth sores or oral ulcers are common with methotrexate. Again, this problem can be reduced by lowering the dosage, giving folic acid along with the methotrexate, and/or using mouthwash treatment.

Despite the list of side effects with methotrexate treatment, it may help to remember that more than 60 percent of people who start methotrexate take it for longer than five years, and more than 40 percent take it longer than 10 years. Low-dose methotrexate is an important, effective treatment for rheumatoid arthritis.

Biologic Response Modifiers

In the 1990s and early 21st century, several new drugs that directly modify the immune system have been introduced to great fanfare and excitement: the biologic response modifiers, a new subset of DMARDs. Early recipients of these drugs often saw dramatic results, causing in one case a temporary shortage of the drug due to demand. This new group includes etanercept (*Enbrel*), infliximab (*Remicade*), anakinra (*Kineret*) and adalimumab (*Humira*).

Biologic response modifiers specifically inhibit chemicals (called *cytokines*) that are involved in the inflammatory response. Etanercept, infliximab and adalimumab inhibit a cytokine called *tumor necrosis factor,* and they are often called *TNF-inhibitors.* Anakinra inhibits another cytokine, *interleukin-1.* These new compounds not only can relieve hard-to-treat symptoms of RA, but they also may inhibit the structural joint damage that arthritis often causes.

As we discussed earlier in the book, no case of rheumatoid arthritis is exactly like another, and no RA patient is identical to another. So despite the excitement associated with these innovative new treatments, you and your doctor will still have to work together to find the particular treatment that works for you over the long-term. In many cases, combinations of new drugs and older, more established treatments still work best.

Etanercept, anakinra and adalimumab can be self-injected by the patient using prefilled devices. Infliximab must be infused by a health-care professional.

BRMs are still quite expensive. Insurance companies and managed-care organizations may be resistant to their use unless a case of the disease was not controlled with another DMARD, because a drug like etanercept may cost at least 10 times as much as most of the other medications for rheumatoid arthritis.

It's clear that BRMs are a major breakthrough in the treatment of RA, so this is an excellent drug to try as an aggressive therapy. With BRMs, total remission may be attained, something not often possible with other drugs. As all of these treatments are very new and expensive compared to non-biologic drugs, consult with your insurance company to make sure these drugs are covered under your policy, and work with your doctor to get coverage if you both feel this approach is the right one for you.

As these new drugs have been used by RA patients for several years, some concerns have arisen about possible cautions. Patients with congestive heart failure (CHF) should not take adalimumab, etanercept or infliximab. Rare reports of lupus (with symptoms such as rash, fever and pleurisy) have been linked to treatment with these three drugs as well. Symptoms resolve when medication is stopped. A neurological disease, multiple sclerosis, has rarely developed in patients receiving biologic response modifiers. Seizures have been reported with etanercept use.

If you are exploring the use of the BRMs adalimumab, etanercept or infliximab, let your doctor know if you have a history (or currently have) one of the following conditions: active infection, recurrent infection, exposure to tuberculosis or a positive skin test for tuberculosis, or a nervous system disorder such as multiple sclerosis, seizure disorders, myelitis or optic neuritis.

ETANERCEPT

Etanercept (*Enbrel*) was the first of the BRMs, an entirely new kind of drug specifically designed to treat rheumatoid arthritis. Etanercept blocks a major component of inflammation known as tumor necrosis factor (TNF). This factor is critical in the inflammatory response. Etanercept blocks the action of TNF to help reduce inflammation.

A new study showed that RA patients taking etanercept and methotrexate in combination allowed significantly more people to achieve clinical remission than those taking methotrexate alone. More studies may reveal more about the usefulness of BRMs like etanercept.

Etanercept is given twice per week as an injection under the skin. In most cases, patients inject themselves, but you can have a relative, friend or nurse do the injection. Side effects are minimal in that etanercept is well tolerated and doesn't interfere with blood counts. There is occasional local irritation at the site of injection.

There's a concern that because etanercept may block the inflammatory response too effectively, its use may make it harder for the body to fight infection. So it's recommended that you not start etanercept if a severe infection is present, and the drug should be withheld if you develop an infection.

Because etanercept and other BRMs are still so new, possible long-term effects are unclear. Theoretically, a person may be more susceptible to cancer after taking this drug, but no evidence has emerged thus far that this is the case. Indeed, there were similar concerns about methotrexate 15 years ago, but they have not proven to be a real problem.

Etancerpt is given in 25 mg doses twice per week, given by subcutaneous (beneath the skin) injection. The drug must be refrigerated prior to use. You will mix the dose by injecting liquid into the vial containing medicine in powder form. Do not shake; instead swirl medication prior to injection. You may inject etanercept into the thigh, abdomen or upper arm.

Possible side effects of etanercept include redness and pain, itching, swelling and/or bruising at the injection site; and upper respiratory infection.

INFLIXIMAB

Like etanercept, infliximab (*Remicade*) is designed to block the action of tumor necrosis factor (TNF) in the body. At this time, infliximab is only approved by the FDA for use in combination with methotrexate.

A new study showed that RA patients taking infliximab in combination with methotrexate had improved bone erosion scores on tests compared to those using methotrexate alone. This finding may mean that the drug can help prevent bone erosion. Still, more tests are needed.

Infliximab is also given as an injection but in a very different way from etanercept. You will receive an intravenous infusion once every one to two months in a doctor's office, specialized clinic or hospital. Infliximab is given in doses based on body weight, and ranges from 200 mg to 400 mg per treatment for most patients. The initial dose is repeated at 2 and 6 weeks and once every 8 weeks thereafter. The drug is infused intravenously (IV) during a 2–hour infusion done in a doctor's office, clinical or hospital. Patients taking infliximab should also be taking methotrexate once a week by mouth or injection.

Possible infusion reactions (occurring during or shortly after the infusion) include abdominal pain, cough, dizziness, hives, itchy rash, muscle pain, nasal congestion, nausea, runny nose, shortness of breath, tightness in chest, unusual tiredness or weakness. With infliximab, as with other BRMs, there is a mildly increased risk of common cold or upper respiratory infections.

ANAKINRA

Anakinra (*Kineret*), is the only biologic response modifier currently available that inhibits interleukin-1, an inflammatory cytokine. Like other BRMs, anakinra is given to ease symptoms of rheumatoid arthritis and prevent joint damage.

Anakinra is given in one daily, 100 mg dose given by subcutaneous (beneath the skin) injection. Anakinra can be self-injected in a traditional, prefilled syringe or through an automatic injector device (*SimpleJect*) available through this drug's manufacturer. Anakinra must be refrigerated prior to use,

and the syringes should not be shaken. Anakinra may be injected into the thigh, abdomen or upper arm.

Similar to other BRMs, anakinra's possible side effects include injection site reactions (usually occurring during the first 4 to 6 weeks of use), including redness; swelling; pain and bruising; runny, stuffy nose; sore throat; headache; low white blood cell or platelet count.

You should discontinue anakinra if you have a serious infection (such as pneumonia) or recurrent infections. Live vaccines should not be taken along with this drug, but the flu vaccine or vaccine for pneumonia (*Pneumovax*) can be safely given.

Serious infections, such as pneumonia, occurred in approximately 2 percent of people taking anakinra. The percentage was possibly higher in those with asthma. If you have a current infection or history of serious infection, inform your doctor prior to using anakinra.

ADALIMUMAB

Adalimumab (*Humira*), is the most recent BRM to be approved by the FDA and released. Like etanercept and anakinra, it can be self-injected. Like other BRMs, adalimumab appears to work well to ease RA symptoms and prevent joint damage. A new study showed promise for the use of adalimumab, in combination with methotrexate, in people with long-standing RA. More studies may reveal more about the effectiveness of this and other BRMs.

If adalimumab is used in combination with methotrexate, the dose is 40 mg once every two weeks, by subcutaneous (beneath the skin) injection. If used without methotrexate, the dose is 40 mg once a week, also by subcutaneous injection. Adalimumab must be refrigerated prior to use, and it comes in prefilled syringes.

Similar to other BRMs, which are injected or infused, possible side effects of adalimumab include redness and pain, itching, swelling and/or bruising at the injection site. It also may carry an additional risk of upper respiratory infection.

Like other BRMs, adalimumab should be discontinued if you have a serious infection (such as pneumonia) or recurrent infections. Do not receive live vaccines while taking this drug, but the flu vaccine or vaccine for pneumonia (*Pneumovax*) can be safely given.

If you are planning to begin taking adalimumab, let your doctor know if you have a history of (or currently have) one of the following: active infection, recurrent infection, exposure to tuberculosis or positive skin test for tuberculosis; or if you have a nervous system disorder, including neurological disorders such as multiple sclerosis, seizure disorders, myelitis or optic neuritis. Patients with congestive heart failure (CHF) should not take adalimumab.

Other Disease-Modifying Antirheumatic Drugs (DMARDs)

While the BRMs have received the lion's share of attention in the health press recently, there are a large number of DMARDs now available to treat RA symptoms, either in combination with methotrexate or alone. Some of these drugs are highly effective for some people with RA, and your doctor may prescribe one of them. Two drugs we will discuss, cyclosporine and leflunomide, are chemical compounds that modify immune function and are often very effective in controlling rheumatoid arthritis symptoms. The others in this class are more traditional treatments that are often still used effectively to treat RA symptoms.

LEFLUNOMIDE

Leflunomide (*Arava*) is another drug that affects the immune response directly by blocking metabolic pathways important to the immune system. Leflunomide is quite effective for people with rheumatoid arthritis, both as a single agent and in combination with methotrexate. The dose of leflunomide is generally the same for each person. The typical dose is 100 mg for three days (a loading dose), and then 20 mg per day thereafter.

Side effects include rashes and gastrointestinal symptoms but primarily, effects on liver function. In theory, this would make combination with methotrexate unlikely because methotrexate also can harm the liver. Research studies, however, have shown that methotrexate and leflunomide can be combined safely.

Although methotrexate is the most widely used DMARD, and many people are now taking some of the newer immune-response modulating drugs, there is still a place in treatment for other DMARDs. These include cyclosporine, hydroxychloroquine, sulfasalazine, injectable gold, penicillamine and azathioprine, which may be used in combination with methotrexate or another DMARD. We will also briefly discuss cyclophosphamide, which is not, strictly-speaking, a DMARD, but is used to treat potentially life-threatening forms of rheumatoid arthritis such as rheumatoid vasculitis.

CYCLOSPORINE

Cyclosporine (*Neoral*) was originally developed to prevent organ rejection in people who received organ transplants. It reduces the immune response through regulatory T cells (see Chapter 2). Cyclosporine can be effective as a single drug for people with rheumatoid arthritis, or in combination with methotrexate.

Your doctor will customize the dosage of cyclosporine for you to get the best benefit and least likelihood of side effects. He or she may increase the starting dosage if there are no side effects on blood pressure and kidney function, and may decrease it in the event that side effects are seen, or when there is excellent control of disease.

Side effects of cyclosporine include upset stomach, nausea, loss of appetite and increased hair growth. The most severe complication of cyclosporine is its effect on the kidneys. Blood pressure, which is regulated by the kidneys, may elevate and kidney function may be compromised. Therefore, your doctor will carefully monitor your kidney function with a blood test and measurement of blood pressure every two weeks at first, and every month or two thereafter. Some studies also suggest an increased risk of cancer with long-term use of cyclosporine.

HYDROXYCHLOROQUINE

Hydroxychloroquine (*Plaquenil*) is an antimalarial drug that is of great benefit to some people with rheumatoid arthritis. This discovery was originally made with a related compound known as chloroquine (*Aralen*). Chloroquine was given to travelers to prevent malaria. Some travelers who took chloroquine also had rheumatoid arthritis, and reported dramatic benefit for their rheumatoid arthritis. Controlled clinical trials of antimalarial drugs for rheumatoid arthritis showed substantial benefit compared to placebo (or sugar pill).

A major barrier to the use of chloroquine was that it caused vision to be impaired in a very small number of patients. It certainly sounds scary to hear about eye complications, but fortunately these are relatively rare and can be detected early and addressed if you get regular eye exams.

Hydroxychloroquine is derived from chloroquine and has a much lower incidence of side effects related to the eye. In fact, one can calculate that the likelihood of serious eye toxicity with hydroxychloroquine is much lower than the likelihood of a person being involved in a motor vehicle accident. This does not mean that these events do not occur, but they should not be a major concern for people with rheumatoid arthritis. However, people taking hydroxychloroquine should have an eye exam at least every year or two.

In general, antimalarial drugs are very well tolerated. There are sometimes gastrointestinal distress and rash, as is the case with almost all drugs. However, there are no problems with blood tests or liver or kidney function associated with the use of antimalarial drugs.

SULFASALAZINE

Sulfasalazine (*Azulfidine*) was synthesized with a goal of treating rheumatoid arthritis. It is composed of two molecular components: one is a sulfa molecule such as found in antibiotics, and the other is a salicylate molecule such as is found in aspirin. Sulfasalazine is far superior to a placebo in clinical trials.

An important barrier to the use of sulfasalazine is gastrointestinal distress. Most people with rheumatoid arthritis tolerate 1–2 grams per day very well, but many people have distress even when doses are raised to 2–4 grams per day. Sulfasalazine is often used in combinations. In fact, the combination of methotrexate, hydroxychloroquine and sulfasalazine has been found to be substantially more effective than methotrexate alone in people who have incomplete response to methotrexate.

INJECTABLE GOLD

Gold injections were the most widely used treatment for rheumatoid arthritis from the 1950s through the 1980s, and continue to be widely used in certain centers. Gold was first used early in the 20th century because it was thought that rheumatoid arthritis might be caused by an infection (see Chapter 2), and gold was recognized to be a somewhat effective treatment for infections before antibiotics were developed. During the 1930s, a French rheumatologist named Forrestier began to use gold injections systematically. His work led to the establishment of injectable gold as the major treatment for rheumatoid arthritis from the 1940s to the 1980s.

Although injections of gold were associated with substantial improvement in about two-thirds of patients, side effects were common. The side effects included rash, kidney problems, blood cell abnormalities and lung problems, requiring discontinuation within a few months in more than one-third of patients. Perhaps as important was that many people who experienced a good response over three months to a year lost this response over time. Within two years, only about one-quarter of people who had begun gold treatment continued it.

Injectable gold is usually given as a 10-mg test dose of *Myochrysine* or *Solganol,* two different preparations of gold, followed by a 25-mg dose and then a 50-mg dose at weekly intervals. If the 50 mg dose is well tolerated, the patient is treated with 50-mg injections every week for 20 weeks. The injections are then given every two weeks, three weeks or even four weeks on a relatively indefinite basis, as long as the treatment appears effective and well tolerated – even if additional medications appear necessary. One problem in the use of gold is that its onset of action is relatively slow – it may take up to three months or sometimes longer to see an effect.

Nonetheless, even after five years, about 10 to 20 percent of people who take gold injections continue to have a good response. The combination of gold with methotrexate has been studied, particularly in Europe, where results suggest it is a valuable combination for certain people.

ORAL GOLD

Oral gold (auranofin, *Ridaura*) was developed in the 1980s as a potential substitute for injectable gold. In clinical trials, it was found to be as effective as injectable gold, but these trials generally involved people with rheumatoid arthritis who had not taken other DMARDs previously and did not have long-standing disease. Therefore, oral gold is still used in people with *early* rheumatoid arthritis, but in long-term rheumatoid arthritis it does not seem as effective as many of the other available drugs. The side effects are similar to injectable gold, but oral gold is better tolerated. It is sometimes used in combination with methotrexate or other DMARDs.

AZATHIOPRINE

Azathioprine (*Imuran*) was the first immunosuppressive drug approved for use in rheumatoid arthritis. It controls the production of cells that account for inflammation. At this time, azathioprine is used most of the time as a supplement to methotrexate

or in people who cannot tolerate methotrexate because of the side effects.

Azathioprine does not appear to be as effective as methotrexate, which hypothetically has a similar mechanism of action. Patients who take azathioprine require monitoring every four to eight weeks for blood counts and potential side effects on the liver. Azathioprine has been used in combination with methotrexate, and a few people showed significant improvement. In most people with rheumatoid arthritis, however, there was no major additional benefit from azathioprine.

PENICILLAMINE

Penicillamine (*Depen* or *Cuprimine*) was first used in rheumatoid arthritis because it binds rheumatoid factor, although how it does this is still unclear. Penicillamine is a little like gold in that it is associated with occasional dramatic responses, but only about 10 percent to 20 percent have satisfactory long-term responses. Most doctors use a "go low, go slow" approach, beginning with 250 mg for a few weeks, increasing by 250 mg every four to eight weeks, up to 1,000 or even 1,500 mg per day as needed.

Although penicillamine leads to dramatic results in a few patients, use of penicillamine, like gold, is limited by side effects in 30 to 50 percent of patients who take it for less than six months. These side effects include rash, inflammation of the kidney, effects on production of blood cells, gastrointestinal distress and, in a few people, a peculiar autoimmune syndrome that resembles lupus (see Chapter

3). Penicillamine has been tried in several combinations but it is not used often in the modern treatment of rheumatoid arthritis.

CYCLOPHOSPHAMIDE

Cyclophosphamide (*Cytoxan*) is another immunosuppressive drug that was used by some rheumatologists in the 1970s in people with severe rheumatoid arthritis. It was effective in many people, but carried a high likelihood of severe side effects, including a risk of sterility, bladder complications and a higher risk of cancer. Cyclophosphamide is a potent *cytotoxic* agent that leads to profound suppression of the immune system, but it is not used except in life-threatening situations, such as a vasculitis that threatens to damage or destroy the heart or kidney. Therefore, cyclophosphamide is rarely used to treat rheumatoid arthritis.

MINOCYCLINE

Minocycline (*Minocin)*, though technically an antibiotic and not a DMARD, is a drug sometimes prescribed for treating rheumatoid arthritis. It is not yet approved by the FDA for this particular use. Side effects of minocycline include dizziness, vaginal infections, nausea, headache and skin rash. People who are sensitive to tetracycline medications may not want to use minocycline.

PROSORBA COLUMN

In addition to drugs, another treatment for rheumatoid arthritis that should be noted here is protein A immunoadsorption therapy, or the *Prosorba* column.

In this therapy, patients have a needle, and then a catheter, placed in each arm. Blood is drawn from one arm, and run through a machine that separates plasma from red blood cells, known as an apheresis machine. The plasma is filtered through a *Prosorba* column to remove antibodies and immune complexes that promote inflammation. The plasma is joined again with the red blood cells, then infused through a catheter into the other arm. The procedure is repeated weekly for 12 weeks.

Side effects of this treatment include chills, flu-like symptoms, nausea or vomiting during the procedure and for several hours afterward. Rheumatoid arthritis may flare briefly after a procedure, but will stabilize. In the best cases, the rheumatoid arthritis will subside for 12 to 18 months. This treatment is given periodically over several months, and may cause a temporary, flu-like illness and, in some cases, a rash that makes it necessary to discontinue treatment.

Combination Therapy

It is now clear that no single drug is likely to be a "magic bullet" to alleviate all the inflammation and pain associated with rheumatoid arthritis. Many different types of inflammatory chemicals and abnormalities can cause inflammation in RA, so it's reasonable to imagine that at least a few different drugs may be required to control the disease process. Because each DMARD works by a different mechanism of action, combining them may increase your ability to control inflammation and prevent joint damage.

Research studies have shown that combining certain DMARDs adds considerable benefit without any need to monitor the combination more than a single DMARD, and with no higher likelihood of side effects. As always, it's important to let your doctor know about any medications you are taking for conditions other than your arthritis.

By now you no doubt recognize that there is no single best drug for all people with rheumatoid arthritis. Each individual is unique, and each of the drugs available for this disease will work better for some people than others. There certainly are some drugs that a much larger proportion of the population will find helpful, but you may find one of the other available drugs best for your own case. Because many people will combine different drugs as their treatment, it's important to recognize that certain combinations will be better for some people, and other combinations better for others with rheumatoid arthritis.

Research and Development: Hope for the Future

There are several promising new drugs and therapies to treat rheumatoid arthritis currently in development and under study. Some of the drugs discussed in this chapter have become available recently, and already are being prescribed for many people with rheumatoid arthritis.

You may hear news about pharmaceutical companies conducting research on treating rheumatoid arthritis, and trying to develop new drugs. Be aware that the process takes time – approval by the federal government's Food and Drug Administration (FDA) for a new drug is the result of years of thorough testing to make sure the drug is safe and effective.

Existing treatments, including drugs used to treat diseases and conditions unrelated to arthritis, may someday be found to have a benefit for peopple with RA as well.

A number of new drugs designed to treat rheumatoid arthritis are in the FDA's approval process now. Some of these drugs include rituximab (*Rituxan*), etoricoxib (*Arcoxia*) and CTLA4-Ig. Rituximab showed promise in a recent study testing the treatment on people with moderate to severe RA.

A recent study conducted at the University of Glasgow in Scotland suggested that cholesterol-lowering statin drugs, such as atorvastatin calcium (*Lipitor*), may be a beneficial treatment for RA. More study is needed to confirm this. Many other treatments are in the earliest stages of research and development at various pharmaceutical laboratories around the world.

You may learn about new or potential drugs on the news, or read reports on the Internet. When you hear that a drug has just been approved by the FDA, you may wish to ask your doctor or other health professional for more information to find out if it is a potential treatment for you.

Drugs Used in Treating Rheumatoid Arthritis

NSAIDS: NONSTEROIDAL ANTI-INFLAMMATORY DRUGS

Note: Possible side effects for all NSAIDs, except where noted, include abdominal pain, dizziness, drowsiness, fluid retention, gastric ulcers and bleeding, greater susceptibility to bruising or bleeding from cuts, heartburn, indigestion, lightheadedness, nausea, nightmares, rash, ringing in the ears, reduction in kidney function, increase in liver enzymes.

Ulcers or internal bleeding can occur without warning, so regular checkups are important. If you consume more than three alcoholic drinks per day, check with your doctor before using these products.

Aspirin
Brand names: *Anacin, Ascriptin, Bayer, Bufferin, Ecotrin, Excedrin Tablets, ZORprin, others*
Dosage: 2,400 to 5,400 mg per day in several doses

Choline and magnesium salicylates
Brand names: *CMT, Tricosal, Trilisate*
Dosage: 2,000 to 3,000 mg per day in 2 or 3 doses
Other possible side effects: Bloating, confusion, deafness, diarrhea

Choline salicylate
Brand name: *Arthropan*
Dosage: 3,480 mg or 20 ml per day in several doses
Other possible side effects: Bloating, confusion, deafness, diarrhea

Diclofenac potassium
Brand name: *Cataflam*
Dosage: 100 to 200 mg per day in 2 or 4 doses

Diclofenac sodium
Brand name: *Voltaren, Voltaren XR*
Dosage: 100 to 200 mg per day in 2 or 4 doses (Voltaren); 100 mg in single daily dose (Voltaren XR)

Diflunisal
Brand name: *Dolobid*
Dosage: 500 to 1,500 mg per day in 2 doses

Etodolac
Brand names: *Lodine, Lodine XL*
Dosage: 600 to 1,200 mg per day in 2 or 4 doses (Lodine); 400 to 1,000 mg per day in a single dose for (Lodine XL)

Drugs Used in Treating Rheumatoid Arthritis (cont.)

Fenoprofen calcium
Brand name: *Nalfon*
Dosage: 900 to 2,400 per day in 3 or 4 doses; never more than 3,200 mg per day

Flurbiprofen
Brand name: *Ansaid*
Dosage: 200 to 300 mg per day in 2 to 4 doses

Ibuprofen
Brand names: *Advil, Motrin, Motrin IB, Mediprin, Nuprin*
Dosage: 1,200 to 3,200 mg per day in 3 or 4 doses for prescription-strength *Motrin*; 200 to 400 mg every 4 to 6 hours as needed, not exceeding 1,200 mg per day, for over-the-counter brands

Indomethacin
Brand name: *Indocin, Indocin SR*
Dosage: 50 to 200 mg per day in 2 to 4 doses for *Indocin*; 75 mg per day in 1 dose, or 150 mg per day in 2 doses for *Indocin SR*.
Other possible side effects: Depression, headache, "spacey" feeling

Ketoprofen
Brand names: *Actron, Orudis, Orudis-KT, Oruvail*
Dosage: 200 to 225 mg per day in 3 or 4 doses for *Orudis*; 150 or 200 mg per day in a single dose for *Oruvail*; 12.5 mg every 4 to 6 hours as needed for *Actron* and *Orudis-KT*

Magnesium salicylate
Brand names: *Magan, Doan's Pills, Mobidin, Arthritab*
Dosage: 2,600 to 4,800 mg per day in 3 to 6 doses
Other possible side effects: Bloating, confusion, deafness, diarrhea

Meclofenamate sodium
Brand name: *Meclomen*
Dosage: 200 to 400 mg per day in 4 doses

Mefenamic acid
Brand name: *Ponstel*
Dosage: 250 mg every 6 hours as needed, for up to 7 days

Meloxicam
Brand name: *Mobic*
Dosage: 7.5 to 15 mg per day in a single dose

Nabumetone
Brand name: *Relafen*
Dosage: 1,000 mg per day in 1 or 2 doses, or 2,000 mg per day in 2 doses

Naproxen
Brand names: *Naprosyn, Naprelan*
Dosage: 500 to 1,500 mg per day in 2 doses for *Naprosyn;* 750 or 1,000 mg per day in a single dose for *Naprelan*

Naproxen sodium
Brand names: *Anaprox, Aleve*
Dosage: 550 to 1,650 mg per day in 2 doses for *Anaprox;* 220 mg every 8 to 12 hours as needed for *Aleve*

Oxaprozin
Brand name: *Daypro*
Dosage: 1,200 mg or 1,800 mg per day in a single dose

Piroxicam
Brand name: *Feldene*
Dosage: 20 mg per day in 1 or 2 doses

Salsalate
Brand names: *Disalcid, Mono-gesic, Salflex, Salsitab, Arnigesic, Anaflex 750, Marthritic*
Dosage: 1,000 to 3,000 mg per day in 2 or 3 doses
Other possible side effects: Bloating, confusion, deafness, diarrhea

Sodium salicylate
Brand name: None, generic only
Dosage: 3,600 to 5,400 mg per day in several doses
Other possible side effects: Bloating, confusion, deafness, diarrhea

Sulindac
Brand name: *Clinoril*
Dosage: 300 to 400 mg per day in 2 doses

Tolmetin sodium
Brand name: *Tolectin*
Dosage: 1,200 mg to 1,800 mg per day in 3 doses

Drugs Used in Treating Rheumatoid Arthritis (cont.)

COX-2 INHIBITORS

Celecoxib
Brand name: *Celebrex*
Dosage: 200 mg per day in 1 or 2 doses or 400 mg per day in 2 doses
Possible side effects: Same as other NSAIDs, except less likely to cause gastric ulcers and susceptibility to bruising and bleeding

Rofecoxib
Brand name: *Vioxx*
Dosage: 12.5 mg or 25 mg per day in a single dose
Possible side effects: Same as other NSAIDs, except less likely to cause gastric ulcers and susceptibility to bruising and bleeding

Valdecoxib
Brand name: *Bextra*
Dosage: 10 mg per day in 1 dose
Possible side effects: Headache, abdominal pain, upper respiratory infection, nausea and diarrhea

ANALGESICS

These are drugs used for pain relief. Other than acetaminophen, these drugs have the potential for dependence if used for long periods of time.

Acetaminophen
Brand names: *Anacin (aspirin-free), Excedrin caplets, Panadol, Tylenol*
Dosage: 325 to 1,000 mg every 4 to 6 hours as needed; no more than 4,000 mg per day
Possible side effects: When taken as prescribed, acetaminophen is usually not associated with side effects

Acetaminophen with codeine
Brand names: *Fioricet, Phenaphen with codeine, Tylenol with codeine #3*
Dosage: 15 to 60 mg every 4 hours as needed
Possible side effects: Constipation, dizziness or lightheadedness, drowsiness, nausea, unusual tiredness or weakness, vomiting

Propoxyphene hydrochloride
Brand names: *Darvon, PC-Cap, Wygesic*
Dosage: 65 mg every 4 hours as needed; no more than 390 mg per day
Possible side effects: Dizziness or lightheadedness, drowsiness, nausea and vomiting

Tramadol
Brand name: *Ultram*
Dosage: 50 to 100 mg every 4 to 6 hours as needed
Possible side effects: Dizziness, nausea, constipation, headache, sleepiness

Tramadol with Acetaminophen
Brand name: *Ultracet*
Dosage: 75 mg every 4 to 6 hours as needed for up to five days; no more than 300 mg per day
Possible side effects: Constipation, diarrhea, dizziness, drowsiness, increased sweating, loss of appetite, nausea

CORTICOSTEROIDS

Note: Side effects may be minimal when corticosteroids are taken short-term or at very low doses. The following side effects are possible for all the following corticosteroids, but are more common with high doses and long-term use: Cushing's syndrome (weight gain, moon-face, thin skin, muscle weakness, brittle bones), cataracts, hypertension, increased appetite, elevated blood sugar, indigestion, insomnia, mood changes, nervousness or restlessness.

Dosage varies greatly based on disease severity. Take the amount prescribed by your doctor.

Cortisone
Brand names: *Cortone Acetate*
Dosage: 5 to 150 mg per day in a single dose

Dexamethasone
Brand names: *Decadron, Hexadrol*
Dosage: 0.5 to 9 mg per day in a single dose

Hydrocortisone
Brand names: *Cortef, Hydrocortone*
Dosage: 20 to 240 mg per day in a single dose or divided into several doses

Methylprednisolone
Brand name: *Medrol*
Dosage: 4 to 160 mg per day in a single dose or divided into several doses

Prednisolone
Brand name: *Prelone*
Dosage: 5 to 200 mg per day in a single dose or divided into several doses

Drugs Used in Treating Rheumatoid Arthritis (cont.)

Prednisolone sodium phosphate (liquid only)
Brand name: *Pediapred*
Dosage: 5 to 60 ml per day in 1 to 3 doses

Prednisone
Brand names: *Deltasone, Orasone, Prednicen-M, Sterapred*
Dosage: 1 to 60 mg per day in a single dose or divided into several doses

Triamcinolone
Brand name: *Aristocort*
Dosage: 4 to 60 mg per day in a single dose or divided into several doses

BIOLOGIC RESPONSE MODIFIERS

Adalimumab
Brand name: *Humira*
Dosage: 40 mg injected beneath the skin every other week in combination with MTX; 40 mg once a week when used alone.
Possible side effects: Redness and pain, itching, swelling and/or bruising at the injection site; upper respiratory infection

Anakinra
Brand name: *Kineret*
Dosage: Injected beneath the skin in daily 100-mg doses.
Possible side effects: Skin reactions, including pain, swelling and redness and the injection site.

Etanercept
Brand name: *Enbrel*
Dosage: Injected beneath the skin in 25 mg doses twice per week, or 50 mg given in two daily, 25 mg doses (separate sites)
Possible side effects: Redness and/or itching, pain or swelling at the injection site

Infliximab
Brand name: *Remicade*
Dosage: Determined by body weight. Drug is infused intravenously in a two-hour outpatient procedure every 1 to 2 months. Only approved for use in combination with methotrexate in rheumatoid arthritis.
Possible side effects: Upper respiratory infection, headache, nausea, coughing

DMARDs – DISEASE-MODIFYING ANTIRHEUMATIC DRUGS – and Others

Note: Minocycline, an antibiotic, is included here, since it has been shown to be effective in treating rheumatoid arthritis. Many DMARDs are used in combination to increase effectiveness and decrease side effects. Comprehensive explanations of cautions are in this chapter.

Auranofin (oral gold)
Brand name: *Ridaura*
Dosage: 6 to 9 mg per day in 1 or 2 doses
Possible side effects: Abdominal or stomach cramps or pain, bloated feeling, decrease in or loss of appetite, diarrhea or loose stools, gas or indigestion, mouth sores, nausea or vomiting, skin rash or itching

Azathioprine
Brand name: *Imuran*
Dosage: 50 to 150 mg per day in 1 to 3 doses, based on body weight
Possible side effects: Cough, fever and chills, loss of appetite, nausea or vomiting, skin rash, unusual bleeding or bruising, unusual tiredness or weakness

Cyclophosphamide
Brand name: *Cytoxan*
Dosage: 50 to 150 mg per day in a single dose; may also be given intravenously
Possible side effects: Blood in urine or burning on urination, confusion or agitation, cough, dizziness, fever and chills, infertility in men and women, loss of appetite, missed menstrual periods, nausea or vomiting, unusual bleeding or bruising, unusual tiredness or weakness

Cyclosporine
Brand names: *Sandimmune, Neoral*
Dosage: 100 to 400 mg per day in 2 doses; dose is based on body weight
Possible side effects: Tender or enlarged gums, high blood pressure, increase in hair growth, kidney problems, loss of appetite, tremors

Injectable gold
Brand names: Gold sodium thiolomate: *Myochrysine;* Aurothioglucose: *Solganol*
Dosage: 10 mg in a single dose the first week, 25 mg the following week, then 25 to 50 mg per week thereafter. Frequency may be reduced after several months.
Possible side effects: Irritation or soreness or tongue, metallic taste, skin rash or itching, soreness, swelling or bleeding of gums, unusual bleeding or bruising

Drugs Used in Treating Rheumatoid Arthritis (cont.)

Hydroxychloroquine sulfate
Brand name: *Plaquenil*
Dosage: 200 to 600 mg per day in 1 or 2 doses
Possible side effects: Black spots in visual field, diarrhea, loss of appetite, nausea, rash

Leflunomide
Brand name: *Arava*
Dosage: 10 to 20 mg per day in a single dose
Possible side effects: Diarrhea, skin rash, liver toxicity, hair loss

Methotrexate
Brand name: *Rheumatrex, Trexall*
Dosage: 7.5 to 20 mg per week in a single dose orally; may also be given by injection
Possible side effects: Cough, diarrhea, hair loss, loss of appetite, unusual bleeding or bruising, liver toxicity, lung toxicity

Minocycline
Brand name: *Minocin*
Dosage: 200 mg per day in 2 doses
Possible side effects: Dizziness, vaginal infections, nausea, headache, skin rash

Penicillamine
Brand names: *Cuprimine, Depen*
Dosage: 125 to 250 mg per day in a single dose to start, increased to not more than 1,500 mg per day in 3 doses
Possible side effects: Diarrhea, joint pain, lessening or loss of sense of taste, loss of appetite, fever, hives or itching, mouth sores, nausea or vomiting, skin rash, stomach pain, swollen glands, unusual bleeding or bruising, weakness

Sulfasalazine
Brand name: *Azulfidine, Azulfidine EN–Tabs*
Dosage: 500 to 3,000 mg per day in 2 to 4 doses
Possible side effects: Stomach upset, diarrhea, dizziness, headache, light sensitivity, itching, appetite loss, liver abnormalities, lowered blood count, nausea or vomiting, rash

For more arthritis drug information, The Arthritis Foundation publishes the book *Arthritis Drugs and More: An A to Z Guide*, available for purchase by calling 800/283-7800, or online at www.arthritis.org.

Chapter 12

Surgical Options:

Opening New Doors

For many people with rheumatoid arthritis, surgery is an important treatment option. In addition to other parts of their long-term treatment, such as drugs, exercise, physical and occupational therapy, and joint protection, surgery can improve function and reduce pain in many joints affected by the disease.

At this time, surgical procedures for people with arthritis are becoming more effective and sophisticated. New technology and advances in surgical techniques, as well as the composition of joint replacement parts, is making surgery a more important area of arthritis treatment than ever before. The development of surgical options for arthritis over the last 35 years is one of the major breakthroughs in helping people remain active and continue to enjoy life after their diagnosis.

People with RA can face surgery at various points in the course of their disease, depending on the procedure. For example, in the early stages of the disease, a synovectomy (the surgical removal of the synovium, or lining of the joint) may be performed when one or two specific joints are affected by inflammation much more than most other joints. In later stages, an arthrodesis or fusion of a joint may greatly relieve pain. If s   of a joint has occurred, a total joint replacement or arthroplasty (most comm

matically relieve pain and improve a person's ability to func

aggressive, early treatment philosophy and prescribe new dru

from occurring, some surgical procedures may become less

now, surgery remains a viable, important treatment option

Let's discuss the main procedures used to treat RA, and

gery. Remember: each person is different. No two people

rience from surgery and rehabilitation. You'll learn here

after the operation – to increase the chances of succe

vide additional resources to explore as you consider

Common Surgical Procedures

In the coming sections, we'll discuss the most important surgical procedures for treating rheumatoid arthritis. Your rheumatologist will refer you to an orthopaedic surgeon to perform your surgery. These physicians specialize in surgical procedures involving bone, joints, and soft tissues surrounding bones and joints. Your orthopaedic surgeon will guide you through preparation, the procedure itself, initial recovery, and your long-term rehabiliation. It's likely that you will also work with a physical therapist (PT) during your rehabilitation.

Here are the most common surgical procedures for rheumatoid arthritis treatment. For more in-depth exploration of joint surgery, read *All You Need to Know About Joint Surgery,* published by the Arthritis Foundation. See the back of this book for more information.

SYNOVECTOMY

The *synovium* is the protective lining of the joint. When one or two joints, such as a wrist or knee, stands out as much more severely involved than other joints, your doctor may suggest a synovectomy. This procedure is designed to remove diseased synovium, and will reduce the amount of inflammatory tissue, which will relieve lling and pain. Synovectomy may slow damage to the joint, but the syn- ow back after several years, n to recur.

ually performed in d may be com-

bined with resection (see p. 116). If inflammation has caused tendons to rupture, then your surgeon may repair and reconstruct these tendons simultaneously to improve function. Tendon rupture is rather unusual except in people with rheumatoid arthritis or cases of injury.

ARTHROSCOPIC SURGERY

An *arthroscope* is an instrument that consists of a very thin tube with a light at the end that a surgeon inserts into the joint through a small incision. Arthroscopic surgery has become more and more common over the last 20 years because it involves smaller incisions than traditional surgery, leading to a quicker recovery in most people. In addition, certain types of repairs can be done more easily through an arthroscope. A recent study questioned the value of some minor arthroscopic procedures as having little benefit, but most doctors still feel the procedure can be useful in arthritis cases.

Arthroscopy allows the surgeon to view the inside of a joint. The arthroscope is connected to a closed-circuit television, allowing the doctor to see inside the joint and estimate the extent of damage. The doctor then has many options, including taking samples of tissue for laboratory analysis, removing pieces of loose cartilage or other tissue that can cause pain, repairing a tear in the cartilage, smoothing a rough joint surface, or removing diseased synovial tissue, as a synovectomy (described earlier). Arthroscopic surgery can hypothetically be performed in virtually any joint, but is most commonly performed in the knee and shoulder.

ARTHROPLASTY OR JOINT REPLACEMENT SURGERY

Of all the types of surgery available for people with arthritis, this is the one you've most likely heard about before. That's because joint replacement surgery is one of the biggest success stories in the treatment of chronic joint diseases like rheumatoid arthritis. Joint replacement surgery – or *arthroplasty* – is the surgical reconstruction or replacement of a joint.

Joint replacement is available for many different joints and is most commonly performed on the hip or knee. Joint replacement surgery has been extremely successful in enabling people who might previously have needed to use a wheelchair to walk and enjoy continued mobility and independence. Joint replacement is recommended most often for people older than age 50, but people whose rheumatoid arthritis developed in childhood or at an early age may require joint reconstruction sooner.

The procedure itself involves removing the damaged joint, resurfacing and relining the ends of bones where cartilage has worn away, and replacing the joint with one of several types of man-made components. The components used are made of metal, ceramic or plastic parts.

There are two different categories of replacement joints currently being used: cemented or cementless. Cemented joints are secured in place during surgery with a special cementing material called methylmethacrylate. Cementless joints usually have a porous surface that is fitted next to the bone. Over time, the bone will grow into the joint and hold it in place without the need for cement. In general, cementless replacements are thought to last longer than cemented joints in most, but not all, people. In addition, they usually lead to better bone *remodeling* (the regrowth of bone around the prosthetic joint) and easier *revision* (replacing the artificial joint), if necessary. However, uncemented joint replacements usually require a longer period of limited weight bearing (such as using crutches or a cane) after surgery. So your decision about using cemented or cementless replacement depends on your lifestyle or occupation.

Unfortunately, joint replacements may not last forever. The cement may loosen over time, or one of the components may break. In the early days of joint replacement surgery, about 30 years ago, the replaced joint might have been expected to last only five to 10 years or so. But improvements in both artificial joints and surgical techniques have expanded the life span to 15 years or even more. Many people can anticipate that a joint replaced at this time may last indefinitely. If the joint replacement breaks down over time, revision arthroplasty is often very successful, and further replacement is not needed.

New surgical procedures are making some forms of joint replacement surgery less invasive, requiring smaller incisions and shorter, easier recovery. Computer-assisted arthroplasty

REPLACEMENT
JOINT

HIP REPLACEMENT

aged joints in the feet is still commonly performed to remove *bunions* in the large toe or *hammer toes* in the other toes. Resection can make walking less painful by removing parts of a bone that causes pressure.

Resection is sometimes used in conjunction with joint replacement – a procedure known as *resection arthroplasty*. However, this type of surgery is rarely used as a primary procedure today, due to the development of more successful types of joint replacement surgery. Resection procedures are only used commonly in the feet.

ARTHRODESIS (FUSION)

Arthrodesis is a surgical procedure that fuses two bones together. Although arthrodesis will limit movement, it is usually done to relieve pain and to increase stability in the ankles, wrists, fingers and toes. It may also be performed in the spine, fusing two or more vertebrae together to stabilize the spine and eliminate pain. In rare situations when joint replacement surgery is unsuccessful, becomes infected or if surrounding structures are extensively destroyed, arthrodesis of the hip or knee can provide another surgical option.

In arthrodesis, the bones forming a joint are joined together, often using bones from the patient's pelvis – or sometimes metallic or plastic hardware – to hold the bones together until they begin to grow and fuse together. The resulting fused joint will lose flexibility, but will be less painful, more stable and often more capable of functions such as pinching fingers or bearing weight.

is on the rise, making the procedures more precise. There is a great deal of innovation and research in this field, so in the years to come, joint replacement surgery will become a much easier enterprise for the person with arthritis.

RESECTION

Resection is a procedure that involves removing all or part of a bone. It was most commonly used years ago to relieve pain and improve function in the hands and wrists in early rheumatoid arthritis, and to protect the tendons from damage. It was often combined with synovectomy. Resection of dam-

OSTEOTOMY

The term *osteotomy* literally means "to cut bone." This procedure was used often in the past when joints were *malaligned,* or did not line up correctly as a result of damage to supporting structures and bone. Osteotomy aims to increase stability by redistributing the weight on the joint. Most surgeons perform osteotomy in the hip or knee to shift the load of bearing weight from areas where the cartilage is damaged to areas that still have cartilage to cushion the load.

Surgeons perform osteotomy by cutting the bones whose ends do not line up properly and repositioning them to improve alignment. Osteotomy is generally performed to support weight bearing in the joints of the legs. Because of better control of inflammation, leading to fewer problems with alignment of joints, and improvements in the results of joint replacement surgery, osteotomies are much less common in the treatment of rheumatoid arthritis at this time. In general, osteotomies are most successful in younger active people who have a good range of motion in the joint, good muscle function and some remaining cartilage around the joint.

What You Can Expect from Surgery

In most cases, surgery for people with rheumatoid arthritis is an elective procedure, which means that it is performed by choice and not because it is medically urgent or because of a potentially life-threatening situation (such as the removal of an inflamed appendix to prevent rupture). Nevertheless, it is undeniably a medically important procedure that may dramatically relieve pain and restore lost function and independence.

Personally Speaking   Stories from real people with rheumatoid arthritis

"We were visiting our daughter and her family in Michigan in our RV, and our grandchildren, ages 4 and 7, wanted to stay overnight with Nana and Grampa. The two children slept with Nana, and Grampa slept up front. During the night, my knee and hip began to hurt real bad. I reached for my rub in the darkness, so as not to wake up anyone. Well, I got my tube and proceeded to rub from knee to my hip. Boy, did I smell good! But I still hurt. Turning on the light, I realized that I had reached for the toothpaste.

"My granddaughter will not let me forget my new arthritis rub!"

That Minty-Fresh Feeling
by Barbara Reynolds,
Holland Patent, NY

DECIDING ON SURGERY

Suppose your doctor has suggested that you may benefit from undergoing one of the surgical procedures discussed above. Most likely, you will have some time to consider your decision and discuss your options with your doctor and with the surgeon. Surgery may seem scary, but it is often the best treatment to help you lead a normal life.

Because elective joint replacement procedures are scheduled in advance, it is possible for you to find out quite a bit about the surgery ahead of time – including any risks that might be involved, how the procedure is done, the expected recovery time and how you can participate. As with all treatments, you should consider the risks as well as the benefits. Some of the risks associated with joint surgery include the following:

• **Anesthesia.** Certain risks are associated with the use of general anesthesia and should be discussed with your surgeon and *anesthesiologist* before the surgery.

• **Blood clots.** These can develop following surgery, particularly if the surgery is in your lower extremities. Blood clots are less common than they once were due to improvements in postoperative care.

• **Infection.** An infection can be introduced into the joint and can jeopardize the success of a joint replacement. In very rare instances, the infection may spread to other parts of your body through the bloodstream.

• **Weight.** Being overweight can slow recovery of a joint replacement in a weight-bear-ing joint by adding stress to it. Excess weight can also cause problems with the surgery itself, as it may make the procedure more difficult and a person more vulnerable to complications such as infection in the incision, lungs and other organs.

In addition to these general risks, a person with rheumatoid arthritis may encounter some particular problems with surgery. The drug program used to treat rheumatoid arthritis often must be adjusted prior to surgery, such as stopping NSAIDs and methotrexate for a week prior to surgery. Sometimes dosages can be lowered. This must be carefully planned prior to surgery to avoid having a sudden flare of disease. Another consideration is the need for multiple surgeries. For instance, an individual may need to have surgery in the foot and ankle before planning to have a total knee replacement, so that rehabilitation will go well.

BEFORE SURGERY

Once you have decided to go ahead with surgery, you will need to make plans for the procedure. Your doctor's office will handle administrative details, such as getting preapprovals for surgery. Many orthopaedic surgeons conduct educational programs concerning surgery, including classes, videos or individualized instruction. Take advantage of these programs – they can be very helpful.

The checklist on the following page provides a list of questions that you may review, some of which you might think about during education programs and discuss with your doctor or other health professionals when you are preparing for surgery. Answers to these questions can guide you both in making a decision to have surgery and in determining what to expect before, during and after the procedure.

Checklist: Questions to Ask Before Surgery

1. Do I understand the procedure? Are there written materials, classes or videos of this surgery that I can review to help me understand it better?

2. Can I talk with someone who has experienced this procedure with this orthopaedic surgeon?

3. Will the surgery be done on an inpatient (a hospital stay) or outpatient basis? If I will be an inpatient, how long can I expect to be hospitalized after surgery?

4. Are there minimally invasive procedures available for the type of surgery I need?

5. What are the risks involved in this type of surgery? How likely are they to occur? Do I have any special risk factors?

6. Will I need to lose weight before my surgery – or to qualify for surgery? If so, can you guide me in this effort?

7. What are the risks if I delay or choose not to have the surgery?

8. Is it likely that more surgery will be necessary? If revision surgery is needed, what will that mean? When might that occur?

9. What improvement can I expect from surgery? Is there any downside to this procedure (for example, loss of joint motion following arthrodesis)?

10. Will I need to stop taking any of my medications before surgery? How long before?

11. Can I arrange to have blood taken from me weeks before surgery so that if I need a blood transfusion because of blood loss during surgery, it can be my own blood (the safest form of transfusion)?

12. How much pain should I expect? How long will it last? How will my pain be treated in the hospital and afterward?

13. What exercise program is recommended before and after the operation?

14. When do I start physical therapy? Will it be in my home or at the therapist's office? Will you refer me to a physical therapist?

15. Will I need to arrange for assistance at home after the surgery? For how long?

16. Will I need any special equipment at home? Do I need to make any modifications in my home, such as installing grab bars or ramps?

17. What limits will there be on my activities – driving, climbing stairs, returning to work, having sex – and for how long?

18. How often will I have follow-up visits? Will my rheumatologist be involved as well?

AFTER THE SURGERY

As with any other component of your arthritis management plan, surgery – or rather, the recovery from surgery – requires your active participation for best results. The procedure itself is merely the first step in a longer process of rehabilitating the joint. The end result is worth the effort. Surgeries for arthritis effectively relieve pain and improve joint function.

There are many types of arthritis-related surgery, and some are more complicated than others, necessitating a longer periods of recovery. For example, the rehabilitation required after knee replacement involves considerably more effort than that after hip replacement surgery, and the recovery from hip replacement is usually much more rapid. In general, your surgeon and physical therapist will advise you to begin mobilizing your affected joint as soon as possible, sometimes even before your sutures heal. Movement should be gentle at first, gradually increasing as appropriate.

Within a few weeks of surgery, you should be able to get back to most of your daily activities. Following joint replacement surgery, recovery may take longer and certain activities may be prohibited for a period of several months. Every person is different; some people restrict their levels of certain activities following surgery according to their own needs. Returning to full-time activities is usually possible within three months of joint replacement.

For any surgery to be successful, you must be serious and committed about your rehabilitation. Rehabilitation of a surgically repaired joint can be tedious at times, but we cannot stress enough its importance in this process. A physical or occupational therapist usually guides your rehabilitation. In some cases, a patient begins therapy in a hospital or postoperative rehabilitation facility, but many attend therapy sessions in an office setting. But only a small part of the rehabilitation is accomplished in a hospital, doctor's or therapist's office. Most of the exercise routine will be given to you to perform at home. It will be your goal to keep yourself motivated and to do your exercises faithfully and regularly. The payoff will be proportional to the amount of work you put into it.

Part Three

Managing Rheumatoid Arthritis:
What You Can Do

Chapter 13

Mind Power:

Getting Mentally Tough

Can you really affect your rheumatoid arthritis – positively or negatively – by having a certain outlook? The answer is yes. The major question is how much – and that probably differs greatly from person to person (like everything else with rheumatoid arthritis).

Exciting findings over the last few years indicate that how you react to the stresses and challenges of living with a chronic disease may have a direct influence on the course of the disease. Equally important, your outlook may influence your long-term ability to keep doing all the daily activities that make you independent and make your life meaningful.

Explore different strategies to help you deal with your arthritis. Every person is different, so some of these techniques may work better for you than others. In this chapter, we will first discuss some ideas of how the mind-body connection works, and why it affects your arthritis. Then we will take a look at some of the techniques that have been shown to be effective self-management tools.

The Mind-Body Connection

In the past, doctors suggested there was something called the "rheumatoid arthritis personality." Some researchers had a theory that rheumatoid arthritis could be considered a *psychosomatic* disease – meaning that it was caused largely by "mental" processes that led to physical disease.

As we now know, this idea was a great oversimplification of a very complicated situation. There is no such thing as a rheumatoid arthritis personality; all types of people get rheumatoid arthritis, and the disease affects different people in different ways. However, there was a germ of truth in the idea. It does appear that the mind plays some role in the disease process in rheumatoid arthritis – and most diseases.

For instance, a person's reaction to stressful events probably has an effect on flares of rheumatoid arthritis in some, if not most, people. Continued stress appears to make it harder to control disease. There is evidence that people with optimistic outlooks and feelings of being in control tend to do better over the long-term than people with less positive feelings about their rheumatoid arthritis. This concept of being in control has become known as *self-efficacy*, and its opposite is known as helplessness. We'll discuss these cornerstones of mental strategies in this chapter.

Why Self-Efficacy Can Help

As you know, rheumatoid arthritis is a chronic, painful condition that can cause stress, frustration and depression. These in turn make the pain worse. This cycle of pain is vicious, but it can be halted or reduced through treatment, and by learning to deal with your pain in positive, constructive ways.

Some people who have rheumatoid arthritis may sometimes believe their situation is uncontrollable and there are no effective solutions to help them, a situation known as helplessness. These feelings may result in anxiety, depression and fear of the future. People may lose interest in daily living and cannot make the effort to learn new skills that could help them manage their pain and stress.

Self-efficacy, which refers to a person's feeling that she or he can master a specific situation, may help people with rheumatoid arthritis considerably. People who have good self-efficacy skills tend to be able to cope better with their disease than those who feel helpless in the face of their constantly fluctuating symptoms.

One important thing to remember about self-efficacy is that it is specific to situations, rather than an overall approach to coping

A Pioneer Course Still Going Strong

The Arthritis Self-Management Program, offered by the Arthritis Foundation as the **Arthritis Self-Help Course**, was first developed in 1979 by researchers Kate Lorig, RN, DrPH, and James Fries, MD. At that time, it was considered a groundbreaking idea to provide people with arthritis not only information about their disease but also skills to help them regain control of their lives. "The whole point of the course," explains Dr. Lorig, "is to help people have more confidence to manage their symptoms and be able to live a better life with their disease."

The program originally included information about exercises, muscle relaxation, joint protection, communication between doctors and patients, and taking medicines. As the course was revised over the years, Dr. Lorig found that the most important aspects were those that helped individuals develop their self-efficacy skills. These skills are now emphasized during the six-week program, along with cognitive pain management and aerobic exercises. The success of the course has spurred the development of other excellent programs that help people cope with chronic pain and learn self-efficacy techniques.

To locate an Arthritis Self-Help Course near you, contact the Arthritis Foundation by telephone at (800) 283-7800, or online at www.arthritis.org. Ask for the office of the Arthritis Foundation chapter nearest you. The chapter staff will be able to guide you to local resources in your area.

with pain and stress. Actually, a layman's term for self-efficacy is confidence. For instance, a person may have a high self-efficacy (or confidence level) for walking around the block but a low self-efficacy for climbing Mount Everest.

The good news is that helplessness may be overcome and self-efficacy skills can be learned. When researchers discovered the importance of optimism and self-efficacy, they began to develop programs and courses to help people with arthritis learn these valuable skills. One of the first of these programs – and still one of the most successful – is the Arthritis Self-Management Program, offered through the Arthritis Foundation as the Arthritis Self-Help Course (see box on the previous page). During the course, participants learn and practice self-efficacy skills that help them manage their disease.

Coping With Stress

Having rheumatoid arthritis increases your physical and emotional challenges. You may feel fear, anger and frustration about your pain or physical limitations. These emotions are normal, and are part of the process your body goes through to make sense of this new situation in your life. Some people are able to experience these emotions and simply move on, but many others who have rheumatoid arthritis find it difficult to deal with the ongoing stresses of chronic disease. Finding ways to reduce and handle stress should be an important component of your self-management plan.

WHAT IS STRESS?

Stress refers to the body's physical, mental and chemical reactions to frightening, exciting, dangerous or irritating circumstances. This can be anything from getting the children to school on time to avoiding a crash on the freeway. Every day we face hundreds of stresses – some big and some small – to which we must make appropriate responses.

When we face stress, our bodies are programmed to respond by releasing adrenaline, cortisol and other hormones into the bloodstream. These hormones increase your heart rate, blood pressure and muscle tension, and induce what has been called the "fight or flight response." This kind of response works just fine most of the time. The stress response can actually be beneficial, particularly during emergencies or in high-pressure situations. However, after a stressful situation is resolved, the body's pace needs to return to normal.

Unfortunately, stress levels in our modern society often remain high. You probably experience daily stress on the job, in traffic or because of your health. If you are unable to release tension between stressful situations, your body may start to respond to every pressure as if it's an emergency. Think of your body as a car: It's unhealthy to "race your engine" constantly. You need to shift into neutral sometimes to save wear and tear on your engine.

When the stress response continues for an extended period, it can wear you down. You may find yourself reaching overload and notice that you are accident-prone or that you are making more mistakes than usual. These are signs that you need to try to relieve some of the stress in your life.

MANAGING STRESS

By using methods that have been developed by clinicians and people with arthritis, and tested by researchers, you can learn to improve your own stress-management skills. The first step is to identify what is causing stress in your life (these factors are called *stressors*). Second, you should try to eliminate as many stressors as possible. The third step is to develop effective coping mechanisms to help you counteract the stresses that you cannot eliminate. Some coping mechanisms that can help you manage stress include progressive muscle relaxation, guided imagery, deep breathing techniques and active problem solving.

Step one: Identifying stressors. Before you can change or manage your stress, you must become aware of what's causing it. Identifying your stressors is a process of personal discovery. Of course, there are universal stresses that affect every person's life, such as moving, changing jobs or having a baby. But in your daily life, other stressors are highly individual. What triggers stress for you may not necessarily bother someone else.

One way to discover what causes you stress is to keep a stress diary. The sample diary shown here is a way to note the things that cause you to feel "stressed out." Review your entries at the end of each week to see if there is a pattern of stress-related events. Some people find that this step alone can be empowering. Indeed, extensive research indicates that the simple act of writing down some of the difficulties can in itself lead to better outcomes.

The physical signs of stress can also provide clues and can be noted in your stress diary as well. These include tiredness/ exhaustion, tense muscles, upset stomach, insomnia, cold sweaty hands, changes in appetite, teeth grinding jaw clenching, and general body complaints such as weakness, dizziness, headache or muscle pain. You should be aware that many of these physical symptoms of stress are also symptoms of arthritis. For example, fatigue, weakness and muscle pain are common in rheumatoid arthritis, especially during a flare. Sometimes it's difficult to tell whether your symptoms are caused by stress or by disease – often it's both, or the same thing.

Your stress diary might also include emotional symptoms. These can range from mild irritability to feelings of depression. Anxiety, nervousness and agitation are also common signs of stress. Try to be as specific as possible, so that you can target the most troublesome areas for you.

Step two: Eliminate the negative. Now comes the challenging part – trying to weed out negative pressures in your life. Obviously, not all negative stressors can be eliminated, and sometimes it's stressful just to think about making changes in your life. For instance, you may feel obligated to honor many family and volunteer duties. It may seem easier to continue doing them than to back out. Others may pressure you not to change. But you need to realize that saying no to a few of these obligations may enable you to feel less stressed and have more energy for the things you really must do or want to do.

Review your stress diary. Are there predictable times during the day or week when you feel particularly hassled? For example, being stuck in rush-hour traffic may disrupt your equilibrium and deplete the energy you need to see you through the day. Brainstorm some options that could make your commute easier. Can you leave for work earlier? Can you carpool or take public transportation? Would listening to your favorite classical music make you feel more relaxed? Now

try taking each problem you've identified and see if you can figure out ways to reduce the stress associated with each.

Carrying out this step may be especially difficult for people who pride themselves on their competency and efficiency. Try to remember that no one is immune to stressful stimuli. Try to adjust your mindset by remembering that the more stress you eliminate, the more productively you will be able to handle the tasks you must do. If you can take a step back and become more objective about your situation, it will be easier to evaluate and deal with stress.

Step three: Develop effective coping mechanisms. A positive attitude can contribute to treating the cycle of stress in your life. This does not mean that simply looking on the sunny side of life can make a serious

Putting Stress in Perspective

You can learn to take a more objective look at the stresses and stress-causing patterns in your life by asking yourself these questions:

- Does this situation reflect a threat that is signaling harm, or a challenge that is signaling an opportunity?
- Are there other ways to look at this situation?
- What exactly is at stake?
- What are you saying to yourself right now? Is it productive?
- What are you afraid will occur?
- What evidence do you have that this will happen?
- Is there evidence that contradicts this conclusion?
- What changes can you make?
- What coping resources are available to you?

problem go away. Rather, it means that if you cultivate the ability to be flexible and learn how to deal with change, you will feel less stress and will be able to function more effectively in dealing with problems.

There are many ways to counteract stress positively. For example, if you find yourself dwelling on your problems, you can learn to refocus your attention on solving them and on positive things you enjoy. Thinking about something you like can help you relax and become less stressed. Also, humor is a wonderful way to relieve stress. Schedule time for play, and become involved in activities that make you laugh.

Another important key is to develop and use support systems. Sharing your thoughts with family, friends, clergy or other good listeners can help you view your problems in a constructive way. A support group of people who have arthritis may provide a valuable

source of both listeners and information on dealing with stress.

When you feel that stress is about to overwhelm you, develop a "safety valve" procedure to let off steam. This could involve writing down your feelings in a journal, taking some time to calm down in a quiet setting, or exercising vigorously (but safely). Above all, try to keep a balance between your work, family and recreation activities. Don't feel that you have to eliminate all your fun activities to conserve your energy for work and/or family obligations. It will just increase your stress and your resentment in the long run. Many people with rheumatoid arthritis find that staying busy and concentrating on something other than arthritis boosts their sense of well-being and helps sustain their spirits during times of pain or diminished activity.

Another positive way to handle stress is to take good care of your body. A foundation

Sample Stress Diary

DATE	CAUSE OF STRESS	TIME	PHYSICAL SYMPTOMS	EMOTIONAL SYMPTOMS
4/18	getting kids off to school	7 a.m.	fast heartbeat, tightness of neck	feel rushed, disorganized
4/18	stuck in traffic	8:30 a.m.	headache, heart beating faster, legs aching	frustrated, angry at being late
4/18	meeting presentation	10 a.m.	fast heartbeat, dry throat, clammy palms	anxious, nervous

of good health is like having money in a bank. You can draw upon it in times of need. Make every effort to eat a balanced diet, exercise appropriately, and get enough rest and sleep. Learn to listen to your body for physical signs of stress: If your head aches or your heart is beating fast during everyday situations, such as when you're driving or cooking dinner, you may be pushing too hard.

LEARNING TO RELAX

The ability to relax can help you relieve symptoms of stress, including tight muscles, fast and shallow breathing, fast heart rate, and high blood pressure. In addition, feeling

Stress Diary

Keep a diary or chart if you can and record the causes of your stress as well as physical or emotional symptoms you experience. Keeping a stress diary can help you learn what causes your stress and how you can avoid it. Photocopy this chart or create your own version.

DATE	CAUSE OF STRESS	TIME	PHYSICAL SYMPTOMS	EMOTIONAL SYMPTOMS

relaxed helps you have a sense of well-being and control, which contributes to your ability to cope with stress. Learning relaxation techniques is not easy, especially if you are in pain.

If you would like to try some simple imagery and relaxation exercises, there are several listed at the end of this chapter. Again, remember that these take practice. Don't expect immediate results. It may be several weeks before you reap benefits from some techniques.

If You Experience Depression

Anyone who develops an illness – particularly a chronic illness such as rheumatoid arthritis – may experience psychological distress. This may manifest itself as feelings of depression and helplessness. Not everyone experiences these feelings, but if you do it is important to recognize them so you can find ways to effectively deal with these types of distress.

DEPRESSION

Everyone feels "down" or "blue" occasionally, and they may refer to these feelings as being depressed. Clinical depression, however, is a severe and prolonged feeling that can hamper your ability to function normally. If you think you may have clinical depression, you should discuss it with a doctor because there are many ways to treat this condition.

It has long been debated whether people with rheumatoid arthritis experience higher levels of depression than others without the disease. The confusion about this issue stems in part from the fact that some signs of depression, such as fatigue and feelings of overall poor health, are also signs of rheumatoid arthritis. This confusion is related to the issue of a "rheumatoid personality," discussed earlier in this chapter, which experts do not believe to be a valid concept. Thus, many of the questionnaires designed to assess depression include "physical" rather than "psychological" problems in people who have rheumatoid arthritis, and may be interpreted to indicate that a person is depressed.

A second issue is whether depression is more common in women than in men. It is true that women tend to have higher scores on depression questionnaires, suggesting higher levels of depression. However, one possible explanation for the phenomenon is that women are more likely to recognize and acknowledge depression, as well as many other health problems, than men. It may be that actual levels of depression are similar in men and women, but there is a "reporting bias" that is picked up by the questionnaire.

Although the debate continues on these issues, it is reasonable that there might be some depression associated with the pain, fatigue, uncertainty and loss of function that people who have rheumatoid arthritis must face. There is the fear of what may or may not happen as the disease progresses – how arthritis will affect your ability to perform normal activities and to live independently. It's important to realize that depression – like arthritis – is not something to suffer through silently. It can be treated: You can talk to a qualified professional about your feelings, and you can feel better and in more control of your life.

HELPLESSNESS

Feelings of helplessness may occur when you are unable to do many of the things you used to do independently, or when you are unable to accomplish as much as you previously were able to do each day. As we mentioned at the beginning of this chapter, self-efficacy skills can be used to offset these feelings of helplessness. Results of studies have shown that people who learn to use self-efficacy skills show improvements in both their mental attitudes and their physical abilities to function.

On the following pages, you'll find some activities that may help you learn to achieve relaxation.

Personally Speaking Stories from real people with rheumatoid arthritis

"**I** wonder if there is a person out there who has some golden years to their credit, has been diagnosed with rheumatoid arthritis, and who hasn't experienced this:

"I'd go into the bathroom housing the same facilities I'd been using for umpteen years, and all of a sudden they're aren't facilities anymore – they're obstacles. The appliance that set the most unique trap for me was the toilet seat, in our household referred to as the 'johnny seat.'

Vanity Works For Me
by Betty Moore, Lukeville, AZ

"Sitting down on it wasn't too much of a problem, even though at times, my knees didn't want to bend as easily as they used to, and I'd land with a thud. It was the process of getting up that was tough, beginning what I termed the 'johnny rock.' Getting up off that booby trap turned me into a contortionist, with my arthritis gnawing at my joints. My mind says, 'OK, I'm ready to get up.' Every fiber in my body told me to stand up. But there I sat. I'd get my hands braced so they could help me force myself up and off. That's where the rocking begins. I'd rock back thinking, 'This time I will push myself up and off this seat.' But somehow, it's like I have a magnet sewn onto my bottom, and the johnny seat is made of steel.

"I feel defeated, and then the ultimate motivation takes possession of me. If I can't get off this seat, I will have to call for help from my husband. All of a sudden, an extra surge of adrenaline flows through my veins, and with a very determined push with the hands and shoulders, no matter the pain, *zap!* I'm standing. Vanity – no doubt about it, it works for me."

ACTIVITY: Deep Breathing

Deep breathing is a basic technique that applies to almost all relaxation exercises. This simple technique is key to mastering the art of unwinding. Here are the steps:

1. Get as comfortable as you can. Loosen any tight clothing or jewelry, uncross your legs and arms. Close your eyes.
2. Place your hands firmly but comfortably on your stomach. This will help you feel when you are breathing properly. When you breathe correctly, your stomach expands out as you breathe in and it contracts in when you breathe out. (Many people breathe "backwards" – they tighten their stomachs when they breathe in, and relax their stomachs when they breathe out. If you're a "backwards breather," take a minute to get yourself coordinated.)
3. Inhale slowly and deeply through your nose to a count of three. Feel your stomach push against your hands? Let it expand as much as possible as you fill your lungs with air.
4. When your lungs are full, purse your lips (as if you were going to whistle) and exhale slowly through your mouth for a count of six. (Pursing your lips allows you to control how slow or fast you exhale.) Feel your stomach shrink away from your hands?
5. When your lungs feel empty, close your mouth and begin the inhale-exhale cycle again.
6. Repeat the inhale-exhale cycle three or four times at each session.
7. Whenever you're ready, slowly open your eyes and stretch.

TIP: Breathing deeply can make you feel light-headed or dizzy – especially when you are tired or hungry. It's a good idea to first practice deep breathing while you are sitting or lying down. Once you get the hang of it, deep breathing can be used anytime, anyplace.

ACTIVITY: Relaxation to Control Pain

BEGINNING PART (excerpted from "Imaginative Progressive Relaxation" technique):

First, take some time to make sure that you are in a really comfortable position. Make a quick check from head to toe to determine whether your whole body is being supported. Adjust any parts that feel uncomfortable. Try not to have legs or arms crossed, but most importantly, do what is comfortable for you.

Now, close your eyes. Become aware of your breathing. Feel the movement of your body as you breathe in and out. Breathe in slowly and exhale. On your next breath, focus on the image of breathing in good, clean air . . . and exhaling all your tensions with your breath out. Allow your breathing rhythm to pleasantly slow down. Feel as though tension is being released each time you breathe out.

MIDDLE PART:

Option 1: *"Pain Drain"* Now, feel within your body and note where you experience pain or tension. Imagine that the pain or tension is turning into a liquid substance. This heavy liquid flows down through your body and out through your fingers and toes. Allow the pain to drain from your body in a steady flow. Now, imagine that a gentle rain flows down over your head . . . and further dissolves the pain . . . into a liquid that continues to drain away. Enjoy the sense of comfort and well-being that follows.

Option 2: *"Disappearing Pain"* Now, notice any tension or pain that you are experiencing. Imagine that the pain takes the form of an object . . . or several objects. It can be fruit, pebbles, crystals, or anything else that comes to mind. Pick each piece of pain, one at a time, and place it in a magic box.

As you drop each piece into the box, it dissolves into nothingness. Now, again survey within your body to see if any pieces remain, and you may remove them if you wish. Imagine that your body is lighter now, and allow yourself to experience a feeling of comfort and well-being. Enjoy this feeling of tranquility and repose.

Option 3: *"Healing Potion"* Now, imagine you are in a drugstore that is stocked with bottles and jars of exotic potions. Each potion has a special magical quality. Some are of pure, white light, others are lotions, balms and creams, and still others contain healing vibrations. As you survey the many potions, choose one that appeals to you. It may even have your name on the container. Open the container and cover your body with that magical potion. As you apply it, let any pain or tension slowly melt away, leaving you with a feeling of comfort and well-being. Imagine that you place the container in a special spot and that it continually renews its contents for future use.

Option 4: *"Leaving Pain Behind"* Imagine that you are dreaming now. Although your body stays in the same position, imagine

that you are gently leaving it. . . As you leave your body, notice that you have also left your tension and pain behind. Pick a special spot to visit, one that brings pleasure and a feeling of well-being. Notice how your dreamlike body feels as you visit this special place. Linger here for a while . . . and when you feel ready, return to your position in alignment with your body. When you open your eyes, retain the freedom from tension and pain, and continue to experience a sense of comfort and well-being.

END PART:

Whenever you are ready, slowly stretch and open your eyes.

Adapted from *The ROM Dance,* a range-of-motion and relaxation program, Diane Harlowe and Patricia Yu, 1992. Published by St. Mary's Hospital Medical Center, Madison, WI. Materials available from The ROM Dance, P.O. Box 3332, Madison, WI 53709. 800/488-4940.

ACTIVITY: Guided-Imagery Smorgasbord

Think of guided imagery as a daydream with a tour guide. By diverting your attention away from stress, guided imagery takes your mind on a mini-vacation. Use your imagination to transport yourself to a more peaceful place. It's up to you to choose where. For some people the most relaxing place is the seashore; for others it's the mountains. Pick your mind's ideal vacation spot, and go there. The following exercise teaches you how to focus on relaxing in your choice of desirable, stress-free locations. Again, have a friend read the exercise to you – or record it yourself and play it back as you imagine.

BEGINNING RITUAL:

Get as comfortable as you can, feet slightly apart, arms resting at your sides. Now close your eyes. Take a slow deep breath in through your nose and slowly exhale through your mouth. Again, take a deep breath in . . . and slowly exhale. Continue to breath slowly and deeply. Notice yourself getting more and more relaxed. Let all your tension melt away.

MIDDLE PART:

Option 1: *"Sea"* Your body is very heavy, at ease and warm. . . Listen to your heart . . . it is beating steadily . . . and regularly. . . As you listen to your heart . . . you feel its beat . . . in your whole body . . . It feels as though you are on a boat . . . on a quiet calm sea . . . with the water lapping against the sides . . .

You're inhaling and exhaling like the waves. . . . They are gently rocking you. . . The rocking continues in your mind . . . and as you rock . . . one after the other the negative emotions are dropping out of you . . . frustration . . . sorrow . . . depression . . . heartache . . . worries . . . resentment. . . You feel serene and content . . .

You feel so wonderful you'd like the whole world to enjoy it with you . . . and out of the depths of your heart rises a great lightness . . . and you feel it flow in a continuous steady stream through your whole body . . . and all the time you feel lighter . . . and lighter . . .

Adapted from the *Arthritis Movement Workshop Leader's Manual*, Arthritis Foundation, Arizona Chapter.

Option 2: *"Pine Forest"* Imagine in as much detail as possible that you are sitting comfortably in a chair or hammock in the middle of a beautiful pine forest. . . Enjoy the fresh, cool, clean, fragrant air. . . What a pleasure it is to breathe! . . . Imagine the gentle, cool breeze as it touches your skin.

You are sitting comfortably, feeling peaceful and calm. . . As you casually look around, you are impressed by the beauty of the tall pine trees with their rich brown bark . . . and graceful feathery green branches. You notice the pinecones on the branches. . . . You watch the leaves of the aspen trees dancing in the wind. The ground interests you with its rich brown dirt covered with pine needles and leaves . . . and its robust, earthy aroma.

You hear birds calling . . . and a woodpecker at work in the distance. . . You notice a small clearing in the forest. The clearing is covered with green grass and beautiful wildflowers of all types and colors. You see butterflies around the flowers. You are at peace in your pine forest, sitting comfortably, feeling relaxed and calm . . . appreciating the wonders of nature . . . and of being alive.

Adapted from the *Multiple Sclerosis Self-Help Course Leader's Guide* by Katalina McGlone, 1984.

Option 3: *"Ocean Beach"* Imagine that you are at the ocean. . . . You are sitting comfortably on the beach under the shade of a large beach umbrella. . . . Feel the warm sand under you . . . and the warm, comfortable air around you . . . and the refreshing, soft breeze blowing through your hair. . . Feel the warm moisture in the air upon your face. . . Notice the smell of the ocean . . . Imagine how beautiful, brilliantly blue the sky is . . .

You're sitting on the beach . . . feeling calm . . . peaceful . . . relaxed . . . comfortable. . . You are watching the waves . . . as they grow and break . . . mesmerized as they go in and out from the shore. . . You can hear the thundering of the waves as they break. . . The only other sounds are those of the seagulls. . .

Notice how peaceful you feel . . . sitting on the beach . . . feeling in harmony with nature.

Adapted from the *Systemic Lupus Erythematosus Self-Help Course Leader's Manual* – Katalina McGlone, 1984.

Option 4: *"Floating in Space"* Imagine you are standing on a mat in front of an elevator. The doors open, you step in and watch the numbers slowly change: 1, 2, 3, 4, 5, 6, 7, 8, 9, 10. The doors open, and you step out into deep, dark outer space. Feel yourself floating weightlessly, drifting, being very light. See the pure, velvety deep blue color of space all around you. Look at the earth, small and green-blue . . . Imagine stars and planets moving past you in the distance. Imagine yourself moving towards a space of diffuse white light, as bright and ethereal as a distant star . . . As you approach this light, it increases in size until you feel yourself surrounded by its glow. Being in the light, you feel that you are bathed in feelings of tranquility and well-being.

If disturbing thoughts or feelings enter your mind as you are in this place, allow them to pass by you, just as you imagine planets and stars passing by you on this voyage. Let these thoughts and feelings fade into the distance, leaving them behind you in the same way that you might imagine a comet disappearing over the horizon.

Enjoy the peaceful feelings of this place. . . Slowly float out of the white light, imagining that it has filled your body and you are carrying it with you. Then float back past the stars and planets through the deep velvety blue-black space to the elevator. Step back in, see the doors close, watch the numbers change: 10, 9, 8, 7, 6, 5, 4, 3, 2, 1. The doors open and you are back on your mat. Feel your body on the mat.

Adapted from the *Arthritis Movement Workshop Leader's Manual*, Arthritis Foundation, Arizona Chapter.

Option 5: *"Memory and Fantasy"* In this relaxation exercise, remember a past experience – or create a new one – with your imagination.

Imagine yourself in an environment where you feel secure, comfortable and relaxed. This can be a place you remember . . . a fantasy you are creating . . . or a mixture of memory and imagination. Simply experience whatever comes to you. Sometimes the environment will change during the exercise, and sometimes it will remain the same.

Place yourself in this environment and note how you are positioned . . . standing . . . sitting . . . or lying down. In this secure, comfortable, relaxed environment, look around you. Take in the panorama of colors, forms and textures. If you are outside or can see outside . . . note the season . . . time of day or night . . . and the weather. Look all around you . . . in front . . . behind . . . both sides . . . above . . . and below you. Look at the sky or ceiling . . . the ground or floor . . . in the distance . . . and up close. Are there other people here? Take in all you wish to see. What sounds come to you? Listen for sounds in the distance . . . up close . . . all around you. From what directions do the sounds come?

In this secure, relaxed and comfortable environment . . . is there anything that you can smell? If something to drink or eat presents itself . . . taste it fully and note its texture in your mouth. Is there anything or anybody you are touching? How does it feel?

How does the environment around you feel physically? . . . Warm or cool? . . . Damp or dry? Do you feel movement in the air? How does it feel emotionally? . . . How do you feel inside in this environment?

Once again, take in the sights around you. . . They may have changed. Note the sounds . . . smells . . . tastes . . . and sights. Focus on emotional feelings . . . the feelings inside.

Adapted from *The ROM Dance*, a range-of-motion and relaxation program, Diane Harlowe and Patricia Yu, 1992. Materials available from The ROM Dance, P.O. Box 3332, Madison, WI 53709. 800/488-4940.

Option 6: *"Water Fantasy"* Imagine that you are immersed in water, perhaps in your bathtub. . . in a lake . . . swimming pool . . . or even a whirlpool bath. Imagine that the water is the perfect temperature . . . just warm enough so that every muscle in your body feels as supple and flowing as the very water itself. Experience the water flowing around and coming into contact with each part of you. As it does this, it melts away deeper levels of tension . . . leaving your whole body feeling cleansed and drained of all tension.

Let yourself stay in this wonderful water for a while, letting go of deeper and deeper levels of tension . . . and allowing yourself to feel more and more relaxed.

Adapted from *The ROM Dance*.

END PART:

(Silence) . . . You may go back to this place whenever you want, simply by sitting quietly and remembering this place in as much detail as possible. . . . Whenever you are ready, move your fingers, wiggle your toes, and come back to this world feeling refreshed and invigorated.

Build up your resistance to stress. Stress can have a negative effect on your body. Taking good care of your body can help you build up resistance to stress. Ways to take good care of your body include:

- eating a balanced diet
- exercising
- avoiding drugs and alcohol
- getting enough rest and sleep
- saving energy by pacing your activities
- accentuating the positive.

Incorporate the relaxation techniques you've learned in this chapter into your daily life and you'll reap rewards. Managing your stress — whether or not you have rheumatoid arthritis — can lessen pain and increase good living.

Chapter 14

Physical Challenges:

Managing the Ups and Downs

Having rheumatoid arthritis can create many physical challenges in your daily life. Although treatments for arthritis have improved dramatically in recent years, dealing with daily morning stiffness or occasional flares can seem daunting. Also, you may wonder what you can do to save wear and tear on your joints.

In this chapter, we will discuss some tips and techniques to help you deal with the physical side of rheumatoid arthritis: acute and chronic pain, as well as the physical limitations that can result from stiffness and joint damage.

Your overall program for managing rheumatoid arthritis contributes to lessening pain, so it's important to commit to regular exercise, balancing activity with rest and respecting your limits. This does not mean that you give in to your pain; rather, you are finding ways to manage it.

Pain for people with rheumatoid arthritis may have several causes that should be recognized, because solving the problem may involve different approaches.

• **Inflammation.** This process causes your joints to swell and become red.
• **Damage to joint tissues.** Damage may be

due to the disease process of rheumatoid arthritis, or from stress or pressure on the joints.
• **Muscle tightness or fibromyalgia.** Inflammation of the joints may lead to muscle weakness or stiffness at times. Some people with rheumatoid arthritis also experience fibromyalgia, marked by widespread muscle pain.

Fatigue and poor sleep – both of which are common in people with rheumatoid arthritis – amplify pain. Feelings of depression or psychological helplessness can lower your pain threshold, making you more vulnerable to pain.

While you are no stranger to pain, it does-n't have to dominate your life. Most people experience good days and bad days. Pain management specialists emphasize that a healthy approach to coping with pain can help you maximize your good days and mini-mize the pain you feel on bad days. Whether dealing with acute pain during a flare or ongoing, everyday pain, you can learn to help yourself by thinking about your relationship to pain and applying some of the techniques in this chapter that appeal to you.

One woman with rheumatoid arthritis said she had learned to remind herself during pain episodes that her body was sick, but her mind was not. By using your mind – to implement relaxation techniques or to organize daily chores more efficiently – you can become your own best ally in managing pain.

What Is Pain?

When your body is injured in any way, the nerves of your damaged tissue trigger the release of chemicals. These chemicals relay messages to your brain, causing the unpleas-ant sensations we call pain. There are many causes of pain, as diverse as trauma and inflammation. Pain may be sharp or dull, chronic or acute, localized (felt in only one or two places) or generalized (felt through-out the body). In rheumatoid arthritis, pain may be caused by *synovitis*, or inflammation of the synovial membrane surrounding the joint. The result is swelling and tenderness.

Individual responses to pain vary widely. What one person can barely feel, another can hardly tolerate. This is one reason your doctor must rely on your reports of pain when examining you and when prescribing pain medications. Pain can be measured on various types of scales, such as a *visual ana-logue scale*, which asks you to rate your pain on a scale of 0 to 10 (or 0 to 100), with zero indicating "no pain" and 10 (or 100) being "pain as bad as it can be." Keeping track of your pain scores over time can help you and your doctor see how your disease is progress-ing and whether your pain medications and coping strategies are working.

THE "GATE" THEORY OF PAIN

Your nervous system plays an important role in how you experience pain. You may have heard reports about people with trau-matic injuries feeling no pain immediately after an accident occurred. Somehow the nervous system blocks the pain signals by producing chemicals called *endorphins* to lead to a good feeling. Other situations can trigger production of endorphins, such as the so-called "runner's high," which describes the euphoria experienced by run-ners during their physical exertion.

So why is it that some pain signals get blocked? According to one theory, known as the *gate control theory of pain*, when pain signals reach the nervous system, they stim-ulate a group of nerve cells that form a "pain pool." Upon reaching a certain level of activity, a virtual gate opens up, allowing the pain signals to proceed to higher cen-ters in the brain. However, the gate can also be closed by certain signals. For example, medications such as morphine and other narcotics act as synthetic endorphins that block the pain signal, so the gate does not open.

Research has shown that, in addition to pain medication, there are nondrug factors that can be used to close the pain gate. Some or all of the strategies listed in the box on this page may help you deal with your pain. Many of them are discussed at greater length in this chapter or the chapters that follow, as well as in *The Arthritis Foundation's Guide to Pain Management,* available by calling (800) 283-7800 or online at www.arthritis.org.

Pain experts now believe that the process of chronic pain may be more complex. People with chronic pain may experience actual physical changes in the various nerves that receive and transmit pain signals, causing pain to continue even when the actual stimulus or cause of the pain (such as inflammation) is not there. So in RA and other chronic diseases, you may have to treat the pain as well as its underlying cause. New treatments, including implants, electronic stimulation devices, and time-released drugs, may help in some cases. But there is a great deal you can do to learn to manage your own pain, including those in the box on this page.

Non-Drug Strategies for Closing the Gate on Pain

- Heat or cold treatments. Usually applied directly to the site of pain; heat may be more useful for chronic pain, whereas cold packs provide relief from acute pain.

- Positive attitude and thoughts. Consciously switching to positive thoughts can distract your brain from feeling pain (see Chapter 13).

- Exercise. Keeping your joints and muscles moving helps improve your general fitness level and can decrease pain.

- Relaxation techniques. You can train your muscles to relax and your thoughts to slow down by using these techniques, which include deep breathing, guided imagery and visualization, among others.

- Massage. When done properly, this method can relax your muscles and help you let go of tension.

- Electrical stimulation. Delivered through a small device called transcutaneous electrical nerve stimulation (TENS), it blocks pain by stimulating large nerve fibers, or by causing the release of endorphins. TENS is usually prescribed by your doctor or physical therapist.

- Topical lotions. These are applied directly to the skin over the painful muscle or joint. They may contain salicylates or capsaicin, which decrease sensitivity to pain.

- Acupuncture. Considered a complementary or nontraditional therapy, acupuncture is the practice of inserting fine needles into the body along special points called "meridians" to relieve pain (see Chapter 17 on complementary and alternative therapies).

- Sense of humor. Many studies have demonstrated that humor can help bolster the immune system and increase the ability to handle pain.

Knowing what narrows the pain gate can help you feel more in control and create your own plan of action to deal with pain. However, you should be aware that, just as certain factors can close the pain gate, others can open it, making you feel more pain. Some of these factors, such as a flare, are beyond your control. But there are other factors that you *can* control, at least in part. These include:

- **Prolonged stress or anxiety.**
- **Obsessing about pain and negative thoughts.**
- **Too little physical activity.**
- **Too much physical activity or exertion.**
- **Overindulgence in alcohol.**
- **Overuse of pain medications.**

WHY "GRIN AND BEAR IT" DOESN'T WORK

There may be times when you think that the best strategy for dealing with pain is to simply ignore it. Although this approach may work for short periods – say, as you override pain in your hands to finish typing a document or ignore hip pain to dance at your friend's daughter's wedding – it is rarely wise to ignore or deny pain for long periods of time. If you are reluctant to admit it to yourself, tell your doctor and request medications, remember that pain is a signal that something is not right inside your body.

Research suggests that chemicals released by your body when you are feeling pain can actually make the inflammation of rheumatoid arthritis worse. The only good thing about pain is that it signals you something is wrong. There is no advantage to feeling pain over long periods. Don't be afraid to take medications to relieve your pain.

Just because others cannot see your pain, does not mean you are not justified in addressing it. If you have concerns about becoming dependent on pain medication, speak to your doctor. Most of the drugs prescribed for pain relief are not addictive, and even potentially addictive drugs usually do not lead to chemical dependence in people who experience severe pain.

Managing A Flare

Although rheumatoid arthritis is a chronic disease, you can have acute episodes of pain and inflammation, known as *flares*. Flares may be seen after infections, or after highly stressful situations. Often, however, it is not clear what triggers a flare. You may have long periods of time when your rheumatoid arthritis is quiet, or in remission. Then, suddenly, the inflammation becomes more active and you have an arthritis flare.

Flares can be alarming, not only because of the pain, but because of their unpredictability. You may feel discouraged or afraid of further damage to your joints. You sometimes wonder whether something you did may have caused the flare.

What can you do to combat these feelings? Remember that you have a range of tools in your arsenal to address pain – from asking your doctor to increase your pain medications, to applying cold packs or practicing deep breathing techniques. Also, remember that flares do calm down. You may want to think about how you will handle the inevitable "bad days" and flares before you experience them. Just as regular fire drills help people deal with real emergencies, preparing for a flare can help you jump into action when it happens.

Discuss a plan of action with your doctor. One possible approach would be to adjust your medications temporarily while the disease is unusually active. This will not only relieve some of the pain associated with a flare, it will also help minimize any damage that may occur from unchecked inflammation.

Be aware that your medications may not control the flare right away, even if your dosages are increased. Or they may only have a limited effect on your flare. Of course you and your doctors should be in agreement about possible increases in your medications, or even additions of new medications at the time of a flare. Many doctors will review such a plan for a flare that can be implemented when needed without permission from the doctor.

Personally Speaking Stories from real people with rheumatoid arthritis

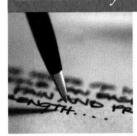

"**I**n 1994, I noticed a strange soreness and stiffness in my hands, then in my wrists and ankles. In less than a year, every joint was engulfed in pain. I found it difficult to continue the simple tasks of living – caring for myself and my family, sleeping, working. They all became almost impossible for me. It hurt just to move. I was living, but I did not feel *alive*. To control the pain, I was on many medications, some with dangerous side effects.

I Call It My Christmas Gift
by Stacy White-Werner, Perry, MI

"Despite medications and therapies, I continued to get worse. Then, in December 1998, I started taking the drug *Enbrel*. I call it my Christmas gift. I have been on this medication since then, and the results are fantastic. I am not in remission, but I am close. I feel stronger every day. I am slowly getting my life back. I am continuing the education that I had put off. I feel like a wife and mother again. When I can completely control my symptoms, I plan on returning to work.

"In addition to medications, I also try to stay active and eat a well-balanced diet. My friends and family are also part of my healing process. Without their love and support, it would be tough to face life with rheumatoid arthritis. They give me the added strength to keep living in spite of it. The other way I cope is by keeping a positive outlook. This is my life, and my body. I'm not going to let rheumatoid arthritis steal any more of it away from me."

The following is a list of some other steps that you may want to incorporate in your plan of action. Remember, some techniques work better for some people than others. Try a few of these, and if they don't work for you, discard them and try others.

• **Balance periods of activity with periods of rest.** Although more rest can help during a flare, you probably do not need to abandon your regular activities, work or exercise program. A doctor or physical therapist can help you modify your program when you experience a flare. Spending long periods of time in bed is counterproductive – it usually will prolong your pain. Instead, try to intersperse periods of rest with some light activity. Finally, to keep joints from becoming stiff, move them through the full range of motion possible, gradually increasing your range as the flare subsides.

• **Have a plan to deal with your obligations.** Have a contingency plan both for work obligations and family obligations. At work, try to arrange for coverage, work fewer hours per week or bring work home. Discuss your plan with supervisors and co-workers ahead of time, and assure them of your commitment. At home, plan to apportion a few extra jobs among family members, and make sure everyone knows what they are expected to do to keep things running smoothly.

• **Communicate with your family and friends.** The time to let your family and friends know that you may need more help is when things are going well. When a flare occurs, if someone volunteers to help you, give them a specific job. Otherwise, well-intentioned offers of assistance go unused. There may be other sources of help available to you as well, such as members of your religious institution or community volunteer organizations.

• **Apply a hot or cold pack to inflamed joints.** Some people find hot or cold packs helpful – different people may prefer one or the other. Although heat can theoretically make inflammation worse, because it tends to increase blood flow and nerve sensitivity, some people find a warm pack soothing and pain relieving. Others get great benefit form cold, which decreases blood flow to the inflamed area and decreases inflammation and muscle spasm. It can provide temporary relief from acute pain. You can buy warm and cold packs from a drugstore or medical supply outlet, or you can use a hot water bottle or simply wrap a towel around a bag of frozen vegetables (to avoid ice burn, never place the ice pack directly on your skin). The pack should be comfortable to the contours of the joint. Leave the pack on the area for about 10 minutes, then remove it for an equal amount of time. Some people even prefer warm packs for certain joints and cold packs for other joints. You will learn your own preferences through trial and error.

• **Practice relaxation or mind-diversion techniques.** These techniques work best when you practice them on a regular basis. Even though relaxation may not directly reduce your pain, it can minimize stress, which is a factor shown to amplify pain.

Many other techniques are available. When you find those that work for you, write them down and use them as often as needed – particularly when you experience a bad day or a flare of your rheumatoid arthritis.

Managing Chronic Pain

Chronic pain – defined as pain that lasts longer than a few months – can be even more challenging to deal with than acute pain. You probably know from experience that a flare does not last, and you will feel

Warming Techniques

- Take a long and very warm shower first thing in the morning to ease morning stiffness.
- Soak in a warm bath or whirlpool.
- Buy a moist heat pad from the drugstore, or make one at home by putting a wet wash cloth in a freezer bag and heating it in the microwave for one minute. Wrap the hot pack in a towel and place it over the affected area for 15 to 20 minutes.
- To soothe stiff and painful joints in your hands, apply mineral oil to your hands, put on rubber dishwashing gloves, and place your hands in hot tap water for 5 to 10 minutes.
- Incorporate other warming elements into your daily routines, such as warming your clothes in the dryer before dressing or using an electric blanket and turning it up before getting out of bed.

A physical therapist can give you many additional ideas for using heat to temporarily relieve pain and ease stiffness.

better. However, handling the chronic pain and stiffness that go on day after day can lead to fatigue, discouragement and even depression. For some people with rheumatoid arthritis, pain becomes a constant companion. It's important to learn to manage your chronic pain, so that you do not become its victim.

Some of the techniques that work for acute flares, such as relaxation, meditation and guided imagery, are also helpful in reducing or minimizing chronic pain. One goal of these approaches is to train your brain and body to focus on positive and pleasing images, thus directing your attention away from your pain. The beneficial effects seem to build over time, so practicing them on a regular basis is important for obtaining good results.

In addition, treatments involving heat or cold can provide soothing relief for stiff joints and tired muscles. There are many forms of these therapies. You can experiment with the warming ideas in the box on this page to find which ones work best for you.

Avoiding Joint Pain And Damage

Managing pain should be proactive, instead of simply being reactive. In other words, you should try to manage pain at its beginning and not wait for it to become severe. Likewise, you can reduce the day-to-day stresses placed on joints in everyday activities to avoid damage.

In addition to regular exercise, you can learn many ways to use your body to reduce joint stress. You can avoid trying to open tight-fitting jars and performing twisting motions on the dance floor. Learning to listen to your body's signals when you need to rest can also reduce pain, because energy reserves can enhance your abilities to cope with pain. Some of the most common techniques are described here, along with examples.

BODY MECHANICS OR ERGONOMICS

Body mechanics is the use of proper techniques for bending, lifting, reaching, sitting and standing. The idea is always to use the largest and most stable joints to do the work. This spreads out the load and lessens stress on weaker joints, or those with more disease involvement.

• **Use your palms.** When you lift or carry things, use the palms of both hands instead of your fingers.
• **Use large muscles.** If you carry a purse, put it over your shoulder or consider switching to a back pack or fanny pack.
• **Lift with your legs.** When lifting something low or on the ground, always bend your knees and lift by straightening your legs.
• **Stand up properly.** To get up from a chair, slide forward to the chair's edge and place your feet flat on the floor. Lean forward, then push down with your palms (not your fingers) on the arms or seat of the chair. Stand up by straightening your hips and knees.
• **Practice good posture.** When standing, practice good posture by imagining a

straight line that connects your ears, shoulders, hips, knees and heels. Knees should be slightly bent, stomach and buttocks tucked in, and shoulders back.
• **Use props.** Put some pillows on a chair, and consider using a raised toilet seat, to help you get up and down more easily.

BALANCING REST AND ACTIVITY

Both work and leisure activities are important – the trick is in balancing them without overdoing it. Moderation should be your motto, especially when your arthritis is more active.

• **Pace yourself.** Take short breaks and alternating heavy and light activities during the day.
• **Don't set unrealistic goals.** Make a "To Do" list that isn't too long – and don't add to it.
• **Keep active.** Too much rest is not good for your joints either. Even on days when you are tired or stiff, try to do some exercise. By increasing your level of fitness, you will actually have more energy and less pain.
• **Know when to take breaks.** Don't wait for the physical signals of pain before you rest.

ORGANIZE AND SIMPLIFY YOUR LIFE

We would all like to be more organized and able to streamline our daily routines. It's an especially good idea if you have rheumatoid arthritis, because the energy you save at work by having everything handy at your desk may mean the difference between coming home exhausted and being able to enjoy the evening. You may expect some guidance from health professionals to help you organize your life, but you can get started by using a few simple ideas.

- **Keep tools handy.** If you work, keep all equipment and tools within easy reach and at a comfortable level. Use a lazy Susan or storage bins to keep supplies handy.
- **Simplify cleaning.** Streamline cleaning chores by using some of the new "all in one" cleaning products, or those that require little or no scrubbing. Don't try to clean everything in one day – rotate the tasks over the course of the week instead.
- **Plan ahead.** When cooking, put all necessary tools and ingredients on the counter before you start to minimize trips to the pantry and refrigerator. Use convenience foods – such as chicken that is precooked and cubed – to save energy and wear and tear on joints.
- **Organize your errands.** If your bank is near the dry cleaner, make one trip instead of two.

SELF-HELP DEVICES

When you're tired, stiff or in a hurry, self-help devices can make tasks easier on your joints and more efficient for you. These products, which range from the simple to the elaborate, help keep joints in the best position for function, provide leverage when needed, and extend your range of motion. The companies listed in the accompanying box are some of the many who sell self-help devices. Simple devices, such as jar openers, reachers and easy-grip utensils can be purchased at many hardware or medical supply stores.

- **In the bedroom.** When dressing, zipper pulls and buttoning aids can help you fasten clothing. Or you can choose to wear clothing with *Velcro* fasteners when available. A long-handled shoehorn extends your reach without bending.
- **In the kitchen.** In the kitchen, appliances such as electric can openers, food processors and mandolins (for slicing) make work easier. Reachers (long-handled tools with a gripping mechanism) can be used to retrieve items stored high or low. Built-up handles and grips make utensils easier to grasp and put less stress on finger joints. Install a fixed jar opener, or keep a rubber jar opener in the kitchen.
- **In the bathroom.** Tub bars and handrails provide additional stability and security when getting into and out of the bath or shower. These are a must if you have problems with balance. Faucet levers or tap turners are available if your grip is weak. A raised toilet seat can make it easier to sit down and get up from the toilet.
- **In the office.** In the work environment, many devices and modifications are available, from adjustable-height chairs and work surfaces to telephones with large push buttons and a special built-up headset. If you are facing work modifications, you will probably want to see an occupational thera-

Where to Purchase Self-Help Devices

The companies listed below are manufacturers of ergonomic office equipment and daily living equipment. You may request catalogs, and may purchase directly from the company or through your physical therapist, occupational therapist or health care provider.

This list is by no means complete, but it may give you a good place to begin searching for useful products. Consult a physical or occupational therapist, or speak to your doctor, to find more sources of self-help or assistive devices. The Arthritis Foundation chapter near you may be able to give you more information on where to find helpful devices, and can give you a copy of the *Arthritis Today Buyer's Guide*, a publication that lists a wide variety of helpful products, services and retailers.

The non-profit Illinois Assistive Technology Project helps people find assistive devices and maintains lists of companies that sell them. This Illinois organization can provide information specific to your state: **Illinois Assistive Technology Project** • 1 West Old State Capitol Plaza • Suite 100 • Springfield, IL 62701 • 800/852-5110 (in Illinois Only) • 217/522-7985 • www.iltech.org

---

ERGONOMIC OFFICE EQUIPMENT
Ergonomic Solutions
129 N. Sylvan Drive • Mundelein IL 60060-4949
(800) 755-4950 • www.goergo.com
Call to obtain their catalog of products, including the Ergo rest and other arm supports, to make computer keyboarding easier.

Ergo Source
P.O. Box 695 • Wayzata, MN 55391
(800) 969-4374
Leave a message requesting company literature to receive their information. Products include office accessories, forearm supports, foot rests and adjustable work surfaces.

DAILY LIVING EQUIPMENT
Smith and Nephew
P.O. Box 1005 • Germantown WI 53022
(800) 558-8633 • www.smith-nephew.com
Upon request, this company will send you their "Activities for Daily Living" catalog.

North Coast Medical
Consumer Products Division
18305 Sutter Blvd. • Morgan Hill, CA 95037
(800) 235-7054
NCM offers a "Return to Fitness" catalog, featuring products for physical therapy and rehabilitation.

Aids for Arthritis, Inc.
35 Wakefield Drive • Medford NJ 08055
(800) 654-0707
www.aidsforarthritis.com
Leave a message with your name and address, and the company will send you their "Self Help Products" catalog.

Sears Home HealthCare
3737 Grader Street, Suite 110 • Garland, TX 75041
(800) 326-1750
Although Sears does not offer a separate catalog for people with arthritis, they will send you a copy of their home health-care product catalog.

Kinsman Enterprises
P.O. Box 364 • Benton, IL 62812
(618) 439-0519
This company deals with hospitals, providers and consumers, and charges the same price to all. Call for their activities of daily living products catalog.

pist. He or she can help you make changes and obtain the devices you need.

• **At play.** Leisure activities can still be enjoyable through the use of assistive devices such as kneelers and light-weight hoses for gardening, "no-hands" frames for quilting or embroidery, and card holders and shufflers for card games, to name just a few.

• **In the car.** When driving, a wide key holder can make it much easier to turn on the ignition. A gas cap opener can help when filling the tank at the gas station.

Chapter 15

Exercise:

The Importance of Getting Physical

If you have rheumatoid arthritis, you may think, "Exercise? Are you kidding? I don't have the energy or ability to even think about exercise!" But exercise is a very important component of RA management, and getting the right kind of exercise can make ordinary mobility easier and less painful.

Perhaps someone has told you that you should rest or protect your joints – and they're right. You do need to take extra care of joints that are actively inflamed. However, that does not mean you should avoid exercise. Believe it or not, it can also be an important way to protect your joints.

In this chapter, we will discuss some of the ways that regular exercise can benefit people with rheumatoid arthritis. We will also review the types of exercises that should be part of your routine, and will even include some simple exercises to get you started.

Why exercise? Some kind of exercise is good for almost everyone, but research has shown that it can be especially helpful for people with rheumatoid arthritis. The disease process – and the damage it causes – may lead to limited joint range of motion, decreased muscle strength and endurance, and general deconditioning. Appropriate and regular exercise can lead to improvement in these areas; it also reduces pain, fatigue and depression. Some researchers have even shown that regular aerobic exercise can reduce joint swelling in people with rheumatoid arthritis.

What if I Don't Exercise?

When you're tired and your body hurts, you may not feel like exercising. It's all too easy to put off exercising because it "uses up energy" you need to complete your other daily activities. However, as the old saying goes, "If you don't use it, you lose

Benefits of Regular Exercise

Keeps your body from becoming too stiff
Keeps your muscles strong
Keeps bone and cartilage tissue strong and healthy
Improves ability to do daily activities
Gives you more energy
Helps you sleep better
Helps control weight gain
Makes your heart stronger and improves cardiovascular health
Provides an outlet for stress and tension
Decreases depression and anxiety
Releases endorphins (your body's natural pain relievers)
Improves self-esteem and provides a sense of well-being

it." Unused joints, bones and muscles deteriorate quickly. Long periods of inactivity can lead to weakness, stiffness, increased fatigue, poor appetite, constipation, increased blood pressure, obesity, osteoporosis, and heightened sensitivity to pain, anxiety and depression. Collectively, these results of inactivity are known as *deconditioning*. And, as the diagram here shows, deconditioning then leads to further pain, in a continuing cycle.

How does the cycle work? If you do not exercise, your muscles become smaller and weaker, and they are less able to support and protect you. You have less stamina and daily activities become more difficult. This loss of function and independence can increase your level of stress, which in turn creates muscle tension, leading to more pain, and so on through the cycle. Exercise is one of the prime weapons used to break this cycle. Luckily, it has been shown that regular exercise actually *increases* the amount of energy you have. Participating in a regular exercise program is a great way to feel better and move more comfortably with less pain.

Making a Commitment to Exercise

The idea of starting an exercise program can be intimidating, particularly if you've never been very active. Just keep in mind that you should start slowly. Do whatever you can at first. As you become stronger and your endurance increases, you will be able to exercise longer and more strenuously.

One of the toughest parts of exercise is just getting started. But the effort you put into starting and maintaining a regular exercise program will come back to you many times over in terms of better health, less pain and improved mental outlook. Once you begin to enjoy the benefits of exercise, your body will become more conditioned, and you will begin to look forward to your workouts.

The following list provides some ideas to help you get started and stay motivated. Use the ideas that make sense for your personality and situation.

• **Get a physical assessment.** See a doctor or physical therapist for an assessment of your exercise and joint protection needs. This will help you understand the reasons for exercise and set reasonable goals.

• **Set realistic exercise goals.** You may even sign a contract with yourself. Write down what you plan to do and when you plan to do it. You could have someone else "witness" the contract to help keep you motivated.

• **Make exercise a routine.** You may try to exercise at the same time each day so that it becomes a part of your routine. Try linking the time to something else: for example, after your morning shower, before lunch or after reading the newspaper.

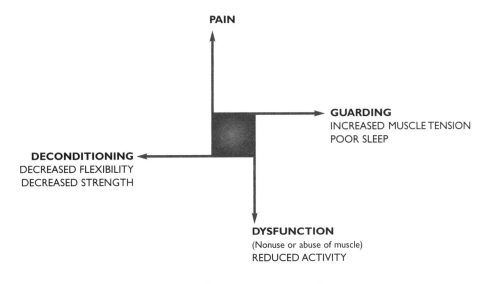

PAIN

GUARDING
INCREASED MUSCLE TENSION
POOR SLEEP

DECONDITIONING
DECREASED FLEXIBILITY
DECREASED STRENGTH

DYSFUNCTION
(Nonuse or abuse of muscle)
REDUCED ACTIVITY

A VICIOUS CYCLE: PAIN, GUARDING, DYSFUNCTION AND DECONDITIONING

• **Stay in the habit.** Do some exercise every day. Extra physical activity can add to improving your physical conditioning. When you feel up to it, incorporate a little extra movement into your normal routines, such as walking up the stairs instead of using an elevator.

• **Make an effort every day.** On days that you have pain or you don't feel motivated, it is important to make some effort – even if you just do some gentle stretching or range of motion exercises.

• **Add variety.** Vary the type of exercises you do to keep from getting bored. Try doing some exercises, such as range of motion or muscle conditioning exercises,

to music. Try rotating other exercises. For example, you could walk three days a week, swim twice and attend an arthritis exercise class twice. Ask a friend or family member to join you in a regular exercise routine. You can help motivate each other, and make exercise something social. If you make it fun, you'll be much more likely to stick with it.

• **Keep track of your progress and enjoy your successes.** There are many ways to monitor the effectiveness of your fitness program. Your doctor or health professional may notice decreased stiffness or improved gait. You will probably be able to see other benefits, such as less fatigue, less pain and decreased stress, for yourself.

The Three Components of Total Fitness

Type	When To Do It	Potential Results
ROM or Flexibility	Every day As needed for better mobility As a warm-up or cool-down	Joint mobility Relaxation Make activity easier
Muscle Toning and Strength	Every other day for each muscle group With flexibility and aerobic exercises	Pain relief More energy Better indurance Make activity easier
Cardiovascular or Aerobic	Every day or as often as possible (at least three times weekly)	More energy Improved weight More stamina Lower blood pressure Better bone health

Choosing the Right Moves

We hope we've convinced you that exercise is important, and important for you. But you may wonder what kinds of exercise you should include in your daily routine. Different people enjoy different types of exercises – and different people with rheumatoid arthritis have different levels of joint involvement, disease course or level of inflammatory activity.

When you are starting out, your first contact may be with a health professional – a doctor, physical therapist, trainer or exercise therapist. He or she may have a list of recommended exercises, and may give you explanatory diagrams. A complete exercise program to improve physical fitness may include exercises for flexibility, muscle strength and endurance, and cardiovascular fitness. How you combine these types of exercise depends on your current capacities, exercise experience, the goals you want to accomplish, and most of all, what you like to do. To become a successful exercise self-manager, you need to discover which types of exercise are best for you and use them to meet your goals.

FLEXIBILITY (STRETCHING) EXERCISES

Flexibility exercises are intended to help keep your muscles stretched out and your joints moving freely. They can be thought of as a foundation of your exercise program, because flexibility is necessary for comfortable movement during exercise and daily activities. It also helps reduce the risk of sprains and strains.

Flexibility exercises are also referred to as range-of-motion and stretching exercises. They should be done gently and smoothly, usually every day. You may be familiar with this type of exercise as a "warm up," because it is usually recommended before performing any more vigorous type of exercise.

If you have been inactive for a while, or if you have stopped exercising temporarily because of your arthritis, these exercises are a good way to begin your fitness program. You can start by building a routine of 15 minutes of flexibility exercises. When you are able to do 15 continuous minutes, you should have the motion and endurance needed to begin adding strengthening and aerobic exercise to your program. Some sample flexibility exercises are included at the end of this chapter.

For people with rheumatoid arthritis, stiffness in the morning can be a big problem. Doing gentle flexibility exercises before getting up or during a hot bath or shower may help joints "loosen up." However, doing them later in the day may be more comfortable for many people with rheumatoid arthritis and may reduce fatigue.

STRENGTHENING EXERCISES

Exercises that increase muscle strength and endurance are the second important component of your fitness program. Joint swelling and pain can weaken muscles, as can disuse due to stiffness and pain. If you have arthritis, strong muscles are needed to climb stairs, walk safely, lift and reach. Strong muscles are important to help absorb shock, support joints and protect you from injury.

Strengthening exercises (also called resistance exercises) make your muscles work harder by adding weight or resistance to movement. There are two types: isometric and isotonic. In *isometric* exercises, you tighten your muscles without moving your joints. This helps build the muscles around your joints. In *isotonic* exercises, you move your joints to strengthen your muscles. For example, straightening your knee while sitting in a chair is an isotonic exercise that helps strengthen your thigh muscle. Flexibility

Recommended Heart Rate Ranges

Age	Heart Rate Range (60% - 75% of Age-Predicted Maximum Heart Rate)	10-Second Count
20	120 – 150	20 – 25
25	117 – 146	19 – 24
30	114 – 143	19 – 24
35	111 – 139	18 – 23
40	108 – 135	18 – 23
45	105 – 131	17 – 22
50	102 – 128	17 – 21
55	99 – 124	16 – 21
60	96 – 120	16 – 20
65	93 – 116	15 – 19
70	90 – 113	15 – 19
75	87 – 109	14 – 18
80	84 – 105	14 – 18
85	81 – 101	13 – 17
90	78 – 98	13 – 16

exercises can become strengthening exercises when you increase the speed, increase the number of repetitions, or add weight (resistance) to the exercise being done.

The goal of a good strengthening program is to "overload" your muscles just enough to get them to adapt to the extra work by becoming stronger. This can be done by adding hand-held or wrap-around weights, elastic bands or simply by using the weight of your body. Avoid loading muscles so much that they are sore and stiff for a day or two after exercising.

If you have active inflammation, or if you feel you need to protect certain joints, check with a therapist about which strengthening exercises are best and safest for you. If you have been inactive, start by doing 15 minutes of flexibility exercises before you attempt any strengthening ones. Some sample exercises are illustrated at this chapter's end.

CARDIOVASCULAR (AEROBIC) EXERCISES

When you hear "aerobics," do you think of young adults in skimpy clothes working up a sweat while loud music blares? Aerobic exercise means more than just aerobic dance. Also known as cardiovascular or endurance exercise, aerobic exercise is any physical activity that uses the large muscles of the body in rhythmic, continuous motions. Walking, dancing, swimming, bicycling or even raking leaves are all examples of aerobic exercise.

These exercises make up the third important part of your exercise routine. The pur-

Finding Your Target Heart Rate

To find your target heart rate, you must stop during your activity and take your pulse. Keep walking or moving around to keep your blood circulating. Placing your index and middle fingers on your opposite wrist or below your jawline at your neck, count your pulse for six seconds and add a zero to that number (or count for 10 seconds and multiply by six). For example, if you count 14 beats in a 10-second period, your heart rate is six times 14, or 84 beats per minute.

Using the chart for a guide, find the target heart rate for your age group. You don't want your heart rate to be faster than the top end of the range during your aerobic exercise. If it does exceed the maximum, slow it down! If you are a beginner, consider the higher number in your range as a "not to exceed" heart rate. And take heart, if you exercise in your target range regularly, your endurance and conditioning will improve.

pose of aerobic exercise is to make your heart, lungs, blood vessels and muscles work more efficiently. This promotes overall health by reducing your risk of heart disease, high blood pressure and diabetes. For people with arthritis, aerobic exercise can help improve endurance, strengthen bones, improve sleep, control weight, and reduce depression and anxiety.

Your fitness program should include some aerobic activities three to four times each week. The goal is to work within your target heart rate for 30 minutes each session. If you are not able to exercise continuously for 30 minutes, work up to it slowly. Start with five minutes of gradually increasing activity, continue with five minutes of activity in your recommended heart range (see chart), then decrease activity for five minutes. Once you are able to do this, you can increase the length of activity in your target range.

Walking. Walking is an excellent type of aerobic exercise for almost everyone. It requires no special skills and is inexpensive. You will need a good pair of supportive walking shoes, and you may need orthotics or special shoe inserts. You can walk almost anytime and anywhere. Many towns now have mall walking clubs, providing a safe place to exercise whatever the weather outside.

Water exercise. Swimming and exercising in warm water are especially good for stiff joints and sore muscles. Water helps support your body while you move your joints through their range of motion. Swimming is highly recommended as an aerobic workout, because little stress is placed on your joints.

Bicycling. Cycling on a stationary bicycle is a good way to get aerobic exercise without placing much stress on your hips, knees or feet. Some stationary bicycles allow you to exercise your upper body as well. When beginning, try not to pedal faster than 15 to 20 miles per hour. As you become more fit you can increase your speed and/or add resistance to your workout.

Rowing. Rowing on a machine – or if you are lucky enough, in a boat – is a good aerobic exercise for people with hip, knee or foot involvement.

Ski machines. Cross-country skiing or using a machine that simulates that action is an excellent nonimpact exercise. It is one of the least abrasive non-water exercises and it works both the upper and lower body.

A Note About Pain

You may be afraid to exercise too vigorously for fear of causing pain or damage to your joints. This is a common concern for many people with rheumatoid arthritis. Thus, it is important to recognize that gentle exercise is best. You can learn to tell the difference between the type of pain you experience from sore muscles after exercising, and the type of pain caused by overuse or inflammation of joints.

Sore muscles are usually the result of overstretching muscles or overusing them when you have been inactive. This type of pain usually begins several hours after exercising and may continue for 24 to 36 hours. If you experience muscle soreness, you may try spending more time doing flexibility or "warm up" exercises before proceeding to more vigorous activity. You may want to scale back your program until your muscles become more accustomed to a certain level of exercise, then gradually increase your workout.

By contrast, swelling and pain may be a signal of overuse of joints. If you notice these symptoms, you can treat the joint by elevating and resting it. You may need to modify your exercise program to avoid further stress to the joint.

One further note about pain: Exercise has been found to be one of the most consistently effective nondrug tools you can use to reduce the pain associated with arthritis. So exercise sensibly, but do exercise. You *will* feel better.

Don't Go It Alone

Many people who exercise on their own find it hard to stay motivated and keep going. If you are among these people, it may help to exercise with at least one other person. Two or more people can keep each other motivated, while joining a class can give you a feeling of shared goals and camaraderie.

Most communities offer a variety of exercise classes, including special programs for people with arthritis, people over 50 or those who need adaptive exercises. The Arthritis Foundation sponsors exercise programs taught by trained instructors and developed specifically for people with arthritis. For information, contact your local chapter or branch office. Programs are also available through local YMCA organizations, health clubs, hospital-sponsored fitness facilities, community colleges, parks and recreation departments, and senior centers.

If you would like to join a community exercise class or health club, try to find one

Personally Speaking Stories from real people with rheumatoid arthritis

"As I sat in the New Orleans airport waiting for my sister to arrive, my heart was pounding. She had been diagnosed with rheumatoid arthritis two months before. The occasion of her visit was her 40th birthday, and I wanted this to be a joyous celebration. But I found myself feeling tearful as I waited for her plane to land. When I saw her, I breathed a sigh of relief. She didn't look any different, just slightly more somber.

Rheumatoid Arthritis From the Outside: A Sister's View
by Beth Hodgens, Macon, GA

"This was five years ago. I was fortunate enough to celebrate my sister's 45th birthday just recently. She came to my hometown to play in a regional tennis championship. She and her partner blew their opponents away in the final match of the weekend.

"My sister is a single parent of two teenage boys, and the director of marketing at a large hospital in Atlanta. Her motto has always been 'Keep moving.' Since her diagnosis with rheumatoid arthritis, there is new meaning in that phrase. Her ability to keep all the balls in the air, her attitude and her movement have helped her gain a handle on her disease. She is a hero to me!"

offering classes that meet your needs. Try to find staff members who are certified by a professional organization, with training or experience in teaching exercise for people with arthritis or other special needs. The facilities should be physically accessible, including the bathroom and changing areas. In addition, you should feel at ease and comfortable with the staff and other members. Let your instructors know your concerns about special needs or modifications. If a facility does not offer you what you need, or you don't feel comfortable exercising there, you may wish to find another one. If you don't enjoy exercising, you probably won't stick with it.

Sample Exercises

Here are some sample flexibility and strengthening exercises that you can try. Note the precautions, if any, and select the exercises that are best for you. You might check with your doctor first before beginning a new exercise program or routine if you are concerned. But most of the time, you are the best person to decide what exercises are best for you. All these exercises are acceptable for some people with rheumatoid arthritis but all are not appropriate for *all* people with rheumatoid arthritis. Use common sense and check with your doctor or therapist if you're not sure.

NECK EXERCISES

Purpose. Increase neck movement. Relax tense neck and shoulder muscles. Improve posture.

Precautions. Do slowly and smoothly. If you feel dizzy, stop the exercise. If you have had neck problems, check with your doctor or therapist before doing these exercises.

I. CHIN TUCKS
Pull your chin back as if to make a double chin. Keep your head straight – don't look down. Hold three seconds. Then raise your neck straight up as if someone was pulling straight up on your hair.

2. HEAD TURNS (ROTATION)
Turn your head to look over your shoulder. Hold three seconds. Return to the center and then turn to look over your other shoulder. Hold three seconds. Repeat.

SHOULDER GIRDLE EXERCISES

Purpose. Increase mobility of the shoulder girdle (the bony structure that supports your upper limbs). Strengthen muscles that raise shoulders. Relax tense neck and shoulder muscles.

Precautions. If the exercise increases pain, discontinue and consult your doctor.

3. HEAD TILTS

Focus on an object in front of you. Tilt your head sideways toward your right shoulder. Hold three seconds. Return to the center and tilt toward your left shoulder. Hold three seconds. Do not twist head but continue to look forward. Do not raise your shoulder toward your ear.

4. SHOULDER SHRUGS (ELEVATION)

(A) Raise one shoulder, lower it. Then raise the other shoulder. Be sure the first shoulder is completely relaxed and lowered before raising the other. (B) Raise both shoulders up toward the ears. Hold three seconds. Relax. Concentrate on completely relaxing shoulders as they come down. Do not tilt the head or body in either direction. Do not hunch shoulders forward or pinch shoulder blades together.

5. SHOULDER CIRCLES

Lift both shoulders up, move them forward, then down and back in a circling motion. Then lift both shoulders up, move them backward, then down and forward in a circling motion.

ARM EXERCISES (SHOULDERS AND ELBOWS)

Purpose. Increase shoulder and/or elbow motion. Strengthen shoulder and/or elbow muscles. Relax tense neck and shoulder muscles. Improve posture.

Precautions. If you have had shoulder or elbow surgery, check with your surgeon before doing these exercises. These exercises are not advised for people with significant shoulder joint damage, such as unstable joints or total cuff tears.

6. FORWARD ARM REACH (FLEXION)
Raise one or both arms forward and upward as high as possible. Return to your starting position.

7. SELF BACK RUB (INTERNAL ROTATION)
While seated, slide a few inches forward from th
back of your chair. Sit up as straight as possible, c
not round your shoulders. Place the back of you
hands on your lower back. Slowly move them
upward until you feel a stretch in your shoulder
Hold three seconds, then slide your hands back
down. You can use one hand to help the other.
Move within the limits of your pain. Do not force

8. SHOULDER ROTATOR

Sit or stand as straight as possible. Reach up and place your hands on the back of your head. (If you cannot reach your head, place your arms in a "muscle man" position with elbows bent in a right angle and upper arm at shoulder level.) Take a deep breath in. As you breathe out, bring your elbows together in front of you. Slowly move elbows apart as you breathe in.

9. DOOR OPENER (PRONATION AND SUPINATION)

Bend your elbows and hold them in to your sides. Your forearms should be parallel to the floor. Slowly turn forearms and palms to face the ceiling. Hold three seconds and then turn them slowly toward the floor.

WRIST EXERCISES

Purpose. Increase wrist motion. Strengthen wrist muscles.

Precaution. If you have had wrist or elbow surgery, check with your doctor before doing this exercise. Stop if you feel any numbness or tingling.

10. WRIST BEND (EXTENSION)

If sitting, rest hands and forearms on thighs, table, or arms of chair. If standing, bend your elbows and hold hands in front of you, palms down. Lift up palms and fingers, keeping forearms flat. Hold three seconds. Relax.

FINGER EXERCISES

Purpose. Increase finger motion. Increase ability to grip and hold objects.

Precautions. If the exercise increases finger pain, stop and consult your doctor.

A)   B)

11. THUMB BEND AND FINGER CURL (FLEXION/EXTENSION)

(A) With hands open and fingers relaxed, reach thumb across your palm and try to touch the base of your little finger. Hold three seconds. Stretch thumb back out to the other side as far as possible.
(B) Make a loose fist by curling all your fingers into your palm. Keep your thumb out. Hold for three seconds. Then stretch out your fingers to straighten them.

TRUNK EXERCISES

Purpose. Increase trunk flexibility. Stretch and strengthen back and abdominal muscles.

Precautions. If you have osteoporosis, back compression fracture, previous back surgery or a hip replacement, check with your doctor before doing these exercises. Do not bend your body forward or backward unless specifically told to do so. Move slowly and immediately stop any exercise that causes you back or neck pain.

12. SIDE BENDS

While standing, keep weight evenly on both hips. Lean toward the right and reach your fingers toward the floor. Hold three seconds. Return to center and repeat exercise toward the left. Do not lean forward or backward while bending, and do not twist the torso.

13. TRUNK TWIST (ROTATION)

Place your hands on your hips, straight out to the side, crossed over your chest, or on opposite elbows. Twist your body around to look over your right shoulder. Hold three seconds. Return to the center and then twist to the left. Be sure you are twisting at the waist and not at your neck or hips. NOTE: Vary the exercise by holding a ball in front of or next to your body.

LOWER BODY EXERCISES

Purpose. Increase lower body strength. Increase range of motion in hip, knee and ankle joints.

Precautions. Check with your surgeon before doing these exercises if you have had hip, knee, ankle, foot or toe surgery or any lower extremity joint replacement. Do not rotate the upper body unless specifically told to do so.

15. BACK KICK (HIP EXTENSION)

Stand straight on one leg and lift the other leg behind you. Hold three seconds. Try to keep your leg straight as you move it backward. Motion should occur only in the hip (not waist). Do not lean forward — keep your upper body straight. NOTE: You can add resistance by using a large rubber exercise band around ankles.

14. MARCH (HIP/KNEE FLEXION)

Stand sideways to a chair and lightly grasp the back. If you feel unsteady, hold onto two chairs or face the back of the chair. Alternate lifting your legs up and down as if marching in place. Gradually try to lift knees higher and/or march faster.

16. SIDE LEG KICK
(HIP ABDUCTION/ADDUCTION)
Stand near a chair, holding it for support. Stand on one leg and lift the other leg out to the side. Hold three seconds and return your leg to the floor. Only move your leg at the top – don't lean toward the chair. Alternate legs.

17. HIP TURNS (INTERNAL/EXTERNAL ROTATION)
Stand with legs slightly apart, with your weight on one leg and the heel of your other foot lightly touching the floor. Rotate your whole leg from the hip so that toes and knee point in and then out. Don't rotate your body – keep chest and shoulders facing forward. NOTE: If you have difficulty putting weight on one leg, you can also do this exercise by sitting at the edge of a chair with your legs extended straight in front and with your heels resting on the floor.

18. SKIER'S SQUAT (QUADRICEPS STRENGTHENER)
Stand behind a chair with your hands lightly resting on top of chair for support. Keep your feet flat on the floor. Keeping your back straight, slowly bend your knees to lower your body a few inches. Hold for three to six seconds, then slowly return to an upright position.

19. TIPTOE (DORSI/PLANTAR FLEXION)
Face the back of a chair and rest your hands on it. Rise up and stand on your toes. Hold three seconds, then return to the flat position. Try to keep your knees straight (but not locked). Now stand on your heels, raising your toes and front part of your foot off the ground. NOTE: You can do this exercise one foot at a time.

20. CALF STRETCH (GASTROC-SOLEUS STRETCH)

Hold lightly to the back of a chair. Bend the knee of the leg you are not stretching so that it almost touches the chair. Put the leg to be stretched behind you, keeping both feet flat on the floor. Lean forward gently, keeping your back knee straight.

21. CHEST STRETCH
(HIP EXTENSION AND PECTORALIS STRETCH)
Stand about two to three feet away from a wall
and place your hands or forearms on the wall at
shoulder height. Lean forward, leading with your
hips. Keep your knees straight and your head back.
Hold this position for five to 10 seconds, then
push back to starting position. To feel more
stretch, place your hands farther apart.

22. THIGH FIRMER AND KNEE STRETCH
Sit on the edge of your chair or lie on your back with yc
legs stretched out in front and your heels resting on th
floor. Tighten the muscle that runs across the front of tl
knee by pulling your toes toward your head. Push the ba
of the knee down toward the floor so you also feel a
stretch at the back of your knee and ankle. For a greate
stretch, put your heel on a footstool and lean forward a
you pull your toes toward your head.

Chapter 16

When You
Feel Exhausted:

Coping With Fatigue

Fatigue is one of the most common symptoms experienced by people with rheumatoid arthritis. Sometimes it is the first sign of inflammation. During periods of inflammatory activity, it is not unusual for people to feel overwhelmingly fatigued, with no energy at all. This overwhelming fatigue can impair your ability to concentrate, make you less able to deal with pain, and increase your feelings of helplessness. Like pain, fatigue is a signal that something is wrong. It is important to pay attention to this signal.

Fatigue may be caused by several different factors including inflammation of rheumatoid arthritis, overdoing routine activities, medication side effects, stress and depression. A lack of restful sleep, poor nutrition and absence of regular exercise also may increase feelings of fatigue.

Feeling tired all the time can lead to a nonproductive cycle of more stress and depression, leaving you less able to meet daily challenges. And, if you become physically run down, your immune system becomes less resistant to infection and illness. In this chapter, we will provide some tools to help you decipher the causes of your fatigue and strategies for managing it. Although some fatigue may be unavoidable, you can eliminate certain sources and triggers of fatigue by being a good self-manager. By setting priorities, making smart choices and conserving your strength, you will still be able to do most of what is important to you.

Pinpointing Causes of Your Fatigue

Your fatigue may be caused by physical, emotional and environmental factors. The box on p. 170 provides a list of some of the more common physical and emotional causes of fatigue, and lists some actions that you can take to address them. In addition to these, environmental factors such as high noise levels, temperature variations, and even daily hassles such as dealing with traffic and waiting in line can make you feel tired.

Identifying the Causes of Your Fatigue

PHYSICAL CAUSES

Are you experiencing a flare of rheumatoid arthritis? The process of inflammation can make you feel tired all over.

Action: Discuss a possible change in your treatment plan, such as increasing dosages of medication to control the flare.

Are you overdoing activities or pushing yourself too hard? Fatigue can be a signal that you are doing too much.

Action: Cut down on the number of tasks you do each day. Learn to alternate periods of activity with breaks.

Have you been doing very little? Too much inactivity leads to muscle deconditioning and can actually make you feel worse.

Action: Incorporate more physical activity into your daily routine (see chapter 15). A therapist can show you safe and gentle exercises that won't harm your joints.

Are you taking any new medications? Fatigue can be a side effect of some medications.

Action: Talk to your doctor or pharmacist about your concerns. It may be possible to switch medications or take them at different times during the day.

Do you awaken feeling rested? If not, you may have insomnia caused by pain.

Action: Your doctor or pharmacist may suggest medications that can ease your pain or help you sleep. Also see tips on getting a good night's sleep in this chapter.

Is your fatigue accompanied by all-over muscle pain or tenderness? If so, you may have fibromyalgia in addition to your arthritis.

Action: Describe your symptoms to your doctor. He or she may prescribe an additional medication, or provide exercise or relaxation tips.

EMOTIONAL CAUSES

Are you experiencing more stress than usual? Your body's response to stress uses up energy, particularly if stress is continuous.

Action: Track your stress using a diary, as discussed in Chapter 13. Prioritize your tasks to conserve energy.

Have you been worrying more lately? It's natural to have worries and concerns, particularly when you have a chronic disease. However, worry drains energy and can become a compulsive habit.

Action: Try using relaxation techniques or sharing your concerns with your spouse or a friend. Write down your worries and then try to find solutions.

Do you feel depressed? People who have clinical depression often experience fatigue.

Action: Seek professional help if you think you may have symptoms of depression. Also, read Chapter 13 for information on dealing with depression.

KEEPING A FATIGUE DIARY

One way to help you discover the causes of your fatigue is to keep a fatigue diary similar to the one shown here. In it, you can note the times of the day or week when you feel fatigue and also what seems to trigger the feeling. Although it may seem like a lot of work, sometimes it's possible to see an obvious solution to the problem that you might otherwise miss. For instance, people often blame themselves for overdoing it when they feel tired, but by reviewing your fatigue diary you may see that your fatigue is actually a sign of increased disease activity that calls for a change in your treatment plan. You may wish to discuss this with your doctor.

A Sample Fatigue Diary

CAUSE OF FATIGUE	POSSIBLE SOLUTIONS
10 a.m. – Parent-teacher conference at school	*Cancel other appointments that day; plan for afternoon rest time*

What Your Doctor Can Do

When fatigue is due to inflammation, it is often more easily corrected than when it is due to stress. The inflammatory cytokines (protein molecules) that are released in rheumatoid arthritis are the same chemicals that are released when you have a severe cold or flu. Although in rheumatoid arthritis they are not fighting to protect your body from disease, they can still leave you feeling weak and tired. Your doctor can improve this type of fatigue by prescribing higher doses of your current drugs or another drug to be used alone or in combination to control the body's inflammatory process. Once inflammation is under control, fatigue usually lessens.

It is also important to consider other potential sources of fatigue that your doctor can reverse. One possibility is anemia, which occurs when the body has too few red blood cells to effectively transport oxygen. A particular type of anemia, often called "the anemia of chronic disease" is often seen in people with rheumatoid arthritis. Effective treatment of arthritis often resolves this type of anemia. Another cause of anemia is due to blood loss from stomach ulcers, and this may require iron replacement and other treatments.

Another consideration is whether the medications themselves are causing fatigue. Fatigue is a side effect of many medications – not usually the drugs used to treat rheumatoid arthritis, but drugs for other conditions such as hypertension (high blood pressure) or depression. Ask your doctor if any med- ications you are taking cause fatigue, and whether any adjustments can be made to improve the situation. Fibromyalgia (see Chapter 5) is also common in people with rheumatoid arthritis, and may cause fatigue.

If you have a second chronic condition (that is, a medical condition in addition to rheumatoid arthritis), your level of fatigue may be even higher. For instance, people with thyroid disease or lung problems often feel fatigued for reasons other than inflam- mation. If you and your doctor address these additional problems, your level of energy should increase.

Sometimes fatigue can be aggravated by not being able to get a good night's sleep. While we will discuss some ways that you can improve your sleep habits, another option is the use of sleeping pills. In some situations, pills to promote sleep can be of great advantage for people with rheumatoid arthritis. Some people have a very good experience with sleeping pills, but others find they don't work well for them. You can work with your doctor to determine the best approach to the use of sleeping pills and which ones might work best for you.

What You Can Do

The most effective approach you can take when dealing with your fatigue is to be aware that fatigue is a part of rheumatoid arthritis, and that you might have to adapt your schedule to the fatigue, rather than fighting it. Don't look at your fatigue as a sign of personal weakness and try to deny it.

It is simply one more symptom of your arthritis that you can learn to handle.

For example, many people with rheumatoid arthritis adjust their daily schedule to start one or two hours later. This makes it easier to deal with morning stiffness and may also enable you to sleep longer. Ultimately, the result is less fatigue and a more productive day. Other people may take a rest or nap in the afternoon, which then allows them to continue with their daily activities without collapsing from fatigue at the end of the day.

Personally Speaking Stories from real people with rheumatoid arthritis

"**W**hen I was 10 years old, my mother was diagnosed with rheumatoid arthritis in an era when not much was known about the disease, and there were no support groups. At 31, I was diagnosed with rheumatoid arthritis also. Naturally, I was devastated, but quickly I learned the value of the Arthritis Foundation and its wealth of guidance and educational material.

My Nine Self-Management Guidelines
by Karen Lenker
Berwyn, PA

"The first step was to choose a physician, one I had good rapport with, for I knew the doctor would be a major part of my life and my friend. I have learned a lot of emotional coping and self-management skills from others. Hopefully, these skills will help someone else, like other people have helped me over the years. They are:

1. Before my feet hit the ground in the morning, I think of 10 things to be grateful for.
2. Exercise in the morning, either walking, riding a stationary bike, or doing exercises or water aerobics at the YMCA.
3. Take time dressing and grooming. Nice soap, cologne, attention to jewelry, or a scarf can perk you up. Most major stores have personal shoppers, and this service can save you lots of energy.
4. Schedule ahead so your days aren't so busy. Include time for rest.
5. Make lists to save time. I always keep a small notepad with me. Doctor's appointments are more productive with a list of subjects to be addressed.
6. Educate family and friends about your arthritis verbally, or with printed material from the Arthritis Foundation.
7. Ask for help ahead of time, so others can put you in their schedules. Sometimes I give a family member a written list to eliminate constant asking.
8. Have fun! Church, hobbies, movies and reading will keep you connected with other people. Support groups are invaluable.
9. Do something for someone else. Help someone in need with an errand, visit or listening ear. Correspond with an old friend or relative. Volunteer."

Using a fatigue diary can help you determine when you feel most tired, and help you adjust your schedule accordingly. Is it right after a heavy lunch? Or do you get sleepy after working at the computer all morning? Try varying your tasks and taking brief breaks to stretch and move around. If you are able, plan to take a walk during your lunch hour a few days a week. Avoid eating heavy meals; instead, opt for a light lunch, perhaps with a healthy morning and afternoon snack thrown in.

Rest is crucial, but it's not the only game in town. It is also important to recognize that doing too little can often lead to deconditioning – which in turn makes you feel more fatigued. Moderate exercise keeps your muscles and joints in condition, and has the added benefit of helping you sleep better at night. There is validity to the conventional wisdom that you get energy by using it!

UNDERSTANDING YOUR BODY'S RHYTHMS

Recent research has shown that people have natural tendencies to be most awake at certain hours and most rested at other hours. These patterns are referred to as your body's *circadian rhythms*. Most people seem to be "morning people" and have their most alert hours in the morning, tend to go to sleep by 9:00 to 11:00 p.m., sleep for seven to eight hours, and awaken between 6:00 and 7:00 a.m. However, some people are "night people" who find it difficult to get up in the morning and feel tired all day if they are forced to get up before restful sleep can occur.

For years, scientists believed that people could change their body's natural rhythms over time, but new findings suggest these adjustments are more complex than first thought. A night person who has to arise before 6:00 a.m. may often feel fatigued all day, unless a nap is possible. Study your own body's natural rhythms, and you may be able to determine the best time to go to sleep and to wake up. Of course, it is impossible to plan your daily schedule completely, but the more you can be in harmony with your natural rhythms, the less likely you will suffer from a high level of fatigue.

GETTING A GOOD NIGHT'S SLEEP

A lack of restful sleep is a problem shared by a great many Americans, and can be due to many different factors. These may include stress; depression; use of caffeine, alcohol or drugs; not allowing enough time for sleep; and pain. When you have rheumatoid arthritis, pain may keep you from falling asleep easily, or it may awaken you during the night. Research has shown that some people with rheumatoid arthritis experience light, easily disrupted sleep with many mid-sleep awakenings. This leads to higher levels of fatigue.

There are several stages of sleep. During the night, your brain moves between these stages in cycles, and the types of electrical brain waves generated vary from stage to stage. To really feel rested, your brain requires what is called "delta sleep," named after the brain waves that occur in the third and fourth stages of sleep. REM (short for rapid eye movement) sleep is also important. It's the stage of sleep when dreaming occurs, and missing it can leave you feeling tired in the morning.

Aging and menopause cause changes in sleep patterns. As people age, there is an increasing variability in the amount and quality of sleep. In older individuals, there is a tendency to spend less time in deep (restorative) sleep and to sleep for shorter periods. Menopause, which usually occurs in the late 40s through early 50s for women, can also cause sleep disturbances such as hot flashes and frequent awakening during the night. Hormone replacement therapy may help alleviate these symptoms.

So, how can you get the sleep you need? Review the checklist on this page for some helpful suggestions, but be aware that it may take time to change your ingrained patterns. If you feel anxious about getting to sleep, you might consider adding some relaxation exercises to your nighttime routine as well.

PRIORITIZING YOUR TIME AND ENERGY

There may be times when you feel more fatigued than others, and you will have to deal with limitations to your energy. Think of your energy as a resource that you have to conserve to have enough for the most important activities. This may involve saying no to lower priority activities that take up too much of your energy.

Of course, it's not always easy to say no, but it helps to stay focused on the priorities

Checklist for Getting the Sleep You Need

Establish Regular Sleep Patterns
- Try to go to bed and arise at the same time each day.
- Avoid taking naps too close to bedtime.
- Take a warm to hot bath within two hours of bedtime.
- A warm non-caffeinated drink may help you relax.

Create a Restful Environment
- Make sure your bedroom is dark, quiet and comfortable.
- Avoid bright light if you have to arise during the sleep period.
- Keep your clock turned away from you.

Exercise
- Exercise regularly each day.
- Avoid vigorous exercise or activity for at least two hours prior to bedtime.

Be Aware of Drug Effects
- Give up smoking, or avoid smoking several hours before bedtime.
- Limit use of alcoholic beverages.
- Cut back or discontinue drinking caffeinated beverages.
- Use prescribed sleep medication only as directed.

Other Considerations
- Avoid large meals two to three hours before bedtime.
- Menopause and aging may cause changes to your established sleep patterns.
- If pain keeps you from sleeping, discuss medication options with your doctor.

in your life, such as earning a living or spending time with your children. When you're feeling fatigued, opting out of an activity may allow you to get the rest you need at this time. Saying no to one activity may allow you to say yes to something more important to you at a later time. Chapter 14 may provide some additional ideas on ways to prioritize your activities and conserve your energy.

ASK FOR HELP, EVEN IF IT'S DIFFICULT

Successful managers are people who have learned that they cannot do everything themselves. Borrowing from their techniques, you can learn to delegate the tasks of managing your activities. Asking for help may be difficult at first. Because the effects of rheumatoid arthritis are not always visible to the outside observer, you may be afraid that co-workers and acquaintances will perceive you as lazy.

You may feel embarrassed to ask for help, especially if you've always prided yourself on being a high achiever. The following suggestions can make it easier to request help from others.

• **Ask for specific help.** For example, if you ask someone to take you shopping for one hour every other Tuesday morning, you are letting them know precisely the help you need. Also, you show others that you understand their time is valuable as well.

• **Develop a "pool" of helpers.** Spreading out the load of additional tasks keeps the burden from falling on any one person. Keep a list of friends and family and which tasks they're willing to help with.

• **Consider bartering or trading services with others.** If you dislike asking for help, perhaps you can provide a service in return. For instance, you can offer to watch your friend's children one afternoon a week at your house, if she will run some errands for you.

Chapter 17

Pushing the Boundaries:

Complementary and Alternative Therapies

One of several messages we hope you have gotten from this book is that there are no easy answers for the complex problems caused by rheumatoid arthritis. Rheumatoid arthritis affects each person individually, making treatment decisions sometimes seem arbitrary. Standard or conventional medicine has no "cures" for arthritis, as it does for infections, stomach ulcers and other diseases.

Because of these reasons, the issue of complementary and alternative therapies has always been a sort of subtext to the treatment program. Study after study has shown that people with arthritis do turn to these therapies, in part due to the fact that drugs do not control disease symptoms completely, and also due to patients' dissatisfaction with the present system of health care. In fact, a 1998 study reported that nearly half of all Americans are trying some kind of unconventional, alternative or complementary therapy. A 2004 British study showed that 44 percent of RA patients surveyed used herbal and OTC treatments.

According to most definitions, an alternative therapy is any practice or substance outside the realm of conventional medicine. Complementary therapy includes practices that coexist with traditional treatment.

Alternative therapies can provide a sense of self-direction and control to people who have chronic health conditions. Some of these treatments, however, fly in the face of accepted scientific principles and natural laws. When accompanied by aggressive or misleading marketing tactics that promise a "cure" for arthritis, many doctors in the past tended to react negatively and refused to discuss these therapies with their patients.

With the establishment of the National Institutes of Health Office of Alternative

Medicine in 1992, now known as the National Center for Complementary and Alternative Medicine (NCCAM), alternative therapies have come out of the closet, so to speak. Many health-care providers realize their patients may try these unconventional remedies and that it is better to discuss such alternatives – and their potential effects – with patients than to ignore the issue.

Learn More About Alternative Therapies

The Arthritis Foundation's Guide to Alternative Therapies ($24.95) offers reliable answers to your questions about nearly 90 different forms of alternative treatments for arthritis, including supplements, acupuncture, tai chi, yoga, chiropractic, meditation, magnet therapy and more. You can order the book directly from the Arthritis Foundation by calling (800) 207-8633 or on www.arthritis.org.

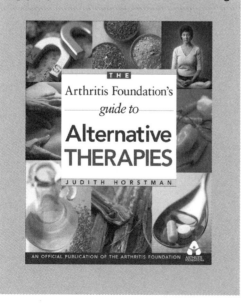

THE
Arthritis Foundation's
guide to
Alternative
THERAPIES

JUDITH HORSTMAN

AN OFFICIAL PUBLICATION OF THE ARTHRITIS FOUNDATION

It would be impossible to discuss the many dozens (perhaps hundreds) of complementary and alternative therapies in a single chapter. Our goal will be to discuss some broad categories of unconventional therapies, then give you information that can help you discuss this topic with your doctor, as well as help you make informed choices about these treatments. The Arthritis Foundation has published a book, *The Arthritis Foundation's Guide to Alternative Therapies*, filled with information on this topic, if you would like more in-depth information about individual therapies.

Types of Complementary and Alternative Therapy

(Note to reader: Relaxation and stress reduction techniques, such as guided imagery and relaxation exercises are discussed in Chapter 13. Exercise is covered in Chapter 15. Although considered complementary therapies, they are recognized as an important part of a comprehensive arthritis management program.)

MASSAGE

Massage therapy is considered by many health professionals to be an excellent way of easing the pain and stiffness associated with arthritis. It can help stretch tight muscles, improve flexibility, and ease pain and stress. Massage is usually categorized as a complementary therapy; in fact, rheumatologists often recommend massage for arthritis and related conditions. Evidence from scientific studies has shown that massage can decrease stress hormones and depression, ease muscle pain and spasms, increase the body's production of natural pain-killing endorphins, and improve sleep and immune function.

Although many different types of massage are available, most include a combination of strokes, friction and pressure that are used to help relax the muscles. Some types, such as Swedish massage, emphasize the physical by using pressing, rubbing and manipulation to work on muscles and joints to improve function. Asian techniques emphasize balancing the flow of vital energy in your body. There are even some techniques – such as reiki and therapeutic touch – that focus on energy for spiritual healing, and practitioners don't physically touch you at all.

What can you expect from your massage? Your session may be given on a padded table or a mat on the floor in a warm, quiet room. It may be softly lit, with quiet music, or it may be more like a typical doctor's office. Before starting, the therapist may talk to you about any special health conditions or sensi-

---

Personally Speaking   Stories from real people with rheumatoid arthritis

"'Energy begets energy' used to be my mantra. 'Movement is life!' my message resounded. Now, the swelling in my joints tells me the truth. Movement is a *gift*.

"I want to exercise. I am sick and tired of my excuses for not being able to participate. Why can't I be the old, energy-packed me? Sure, my excuses are real. I am in my fifth year of rheumatoid arthritis. I have tried to cope with it and accept it. The flares are crippling and strike with no apparent reason. One day I am feeling well, the next day I have hot liquid burning in my joints. Cortisone injections punctured into the offending joints are my only relief.

The Other Side Of Fitness
by Meredith Bunting,
Virginia Beach, VA

"I walk with swollen, cramped feet to greet members in the health club I have managed for 10 years. I direct them to the exercise equipment, and tell them about various energy-packed fitness classes – the ones I used to teach. As they press on to chosen activities, I slip back behind my wall of memories.

"On their way to exercise, my friends greet me. Their smiles touch me like rays of sunshine dispersing murky clouds. They treat me as if nothing has changed. Oh, they know I have had a 'setback.' But they believe in me. They don't pity me. They offer help and lend a hand. I begin to see another side of fitness. It is compassion in action.

"As I accept their help, I sense my walls crumbling. Letting go of what I can no longer do, and inspired by the helping spirit of my friends, I feel a new source of energy. This side of fitness has great potential!"

tivities (such as actively inflamed or painful joints), and discuss your goals for the session. You do not have to remove all of your clothes; often, the therapist will cover you with a large sheet and will uncover only the part of your body that is being massaged.

Sessions vary in length from about 45 minutes to an hour and a half, and cost from $50 to $100 per hour (although prices vary by location and expertise of the therapist). During that time, the therapist will periodically ask how you are or tell you what to do. You should speak up at any time if you feel pain or discomfort, or if you have questions. After the session, most people feel relaxed but energized. Any soreness you feel from the massage should disappear by the next day. If it does not, discuss it with your therapist before the next session.

Although massage is beneficial for many people, it is best to use caution before seeking out a therapist. Therapists may not have experience in participating in the care of people with rheumatoid arthritis, and may not understand their physical needs. Some elements of massage may not be appropriate for people with rheumatoid arthritis. It is best not to have an inflamed joint massaged; in fact, it may make the joint feel worse. Finally, be aware that massage may not be covered by your insurance policy, even when suggested by your doctor.

ACUPUNCTURE/ACUPRESSURE

Long a cornerstone of Chinese medicine, *acupuncture* has been making its way to the Western world for the treatment of many chronic conditions, including arthritis. In acupuncture, disposable stainless steel needles are used to stimulate specific points – located in energy pathways called *meridians* – throughout the body. These pathways have no counterpart in conventional medicine and anatomy.

More than 15 million Americans have used acupuncture, primarily for pain relief. Acupuncture has been used to treat many kinds of arthritis, including rheumatoid arthritis. Some studies have suggested that acupuncture may lessen pain by causing the body to release *endorphins* (naturally produced chemicals that block pain messages and prevent them from reaching the brain). There have also been suggestions that acupuncture has anti-inflammatory effects, but further research is needed to document these phenomena. You are the best judge of whether or not acupuncture is helpful to you.

Acupuncture sessions usually last from 30 minutes to one hour (longer on your first visit) and may cost up to $75 per session. You will be asked to sit or lie on a padded table, to remove or loosen clothing, and to get comfortable before treatment starts. A traditional Chinese acupuncture practitioner may ask you many questions about your health, diet and sleep habits. For the treatment itself, the practitioner will use from two to 15 thin needles, which are inserted at specific points that relate to your condition in Chinese medicine. This treatment may be combined with heat or gentle electrical stimulation.

You should not feel pain, although you may experience slight discomfort when the needles are inserted. The acupuncturist will leave you resting with the needles in place for a short period (20 minutes is typical). Once the needles are removed, you will rest quietly for a while before getting up.

Although the World Health Organization has endorsed the use of acupuncture to treat rheumatoid arthritis, many studies have failed to document the effectiveness of this therapy. If you decide to try acupuncture, find a practitioner who is certified or licensed. Some health insurers will cover these treatments if they are prescribed by (or performed by) a doctor. In addition, make sure that the practitioner uses only sterile, disposable needles.

The idea of having someone insert needles into your body may not seem appealing to everyone. Many people get some of the same benefits from *acupressure*, which is an even older form of this therapy. Instead of needles, practitioners use their fingers or other tools to apply pressure to the same points used in acupuncture.

SPECIAL DIETS OR DIETARY CHANGES

The myth of the miracle arthritis diet is one of the oldest touted alternative therapies. However, scientific studies have never shown that any specific diet alone can control any form of arthritis, with the exception of gout. However, it is undeniably true that your diet affects your *overall* health, and what we eat has been shown to play a role in many disor-

ders. In addition, several research studies indicate that some people with rheumatoid arthritis regularly find that some foods make their symptoms better and others make their symptoms worse. No consistent patterns were identified with all patients.

Ways in which diet might affect your arthritis include the following:

• **Food sensitivities.** A small number of people with arthritis might be sensitive to certain foods that could trigger symptoms or cause them to worsen.
• **Saturated fats.** A diet high in saturated fats or vegetable oils can increase the inflammatory response, thereby contributing to joint and tissue inflammation.
• **Overall health.** Diet affects your overall health, as well as affecting any other diseases or conditions you may have (such as diabetes or heart disease). This, in turn, may affect how your body handles arthritis symptoms.
• **Poor nutrition.** Finally, just having arthritis can make your diet worse. How? You may be unable to shop for and prepare nutritious food for yourself. Pain and fatigue can diminish your appetite, or make it difficult to eat, prepare and chew.

There are many fad diets that claim to alleviate arthritis – everything from fasting to elimination diets (that is, eliminating a certain food or food group from your diet, such as dairy products). The few well-structured research studies concerning diet indicate that what seems to work for one person with rheumatoid arthritis may not work for another. So don't try any extreme dietary changes. If you notice that eating some food makes your arthritis better or worse, don't be afraid to study the situation and act on it.

Your best nutritional bet is to eat the kind of diet recommended by the American Heart Association or the American Cancer Society – one that is low in saturated fats and calories and rich in fruits, vegetables and grains. If you would like to improve or change your diet, consider consulting a registered dietitian. A dietitian can help you change your eating habits, whether your goal is to eat more nutritiously, gain or lose weight, or find out how to prepare easy meals and snacks. The usual fee is about $75 for a one-hour consultation, which may be covered by your insurance. But the real change is up to you – no health professional can control what you eat.

HERBS, SUPPLEMENTS AND "NATURAL" REMEDIES

When it comes to alternative therapies, this category is the largest by far. Supplements such as herbs, minerals, animal extracts and enzymes – as well as more exotic remedies – are increasingly available to people with chronic health problems such as arthritis. What's more, people are buying and using them in record numbers. In 2004, a U.S. government study reported that 19 percent of U.S. adults use natural supplements.

Herbs, supplements and other such "natural" remedies have a tremendous attraction

for people with arthritis who are frustrated with the solutions offered by conventional medicine. Although most people realize there is no "magic bullet" to cure arthritis, they hope their pain and other symptoms will be better controlled if they try a supplement or extract in addition to their formally prescribed medication.

Supplements offer the convenience of popping a pill or potion along with the premise that the "natural" ingredients won't harm you. But natural doesn't always mean safe. Some people think that supplements – especially herbs – are safe because they are natural alternatives to the chemicals used in prescription drugs. The fact is, herbs *are* chemicals. And anything that's strong enough to help may also be strong enough to hurt.

All this is not to say that supplements are not good. In fact, certain types of extracts and supplements have been shown to be useful in treating various types of arthritis. For example, the omega-3 fatty acids found in the oils from certain fish have been shown to modify inflammation associated with rheumatoid arthritis when taken in large quantities. Unfortunately, the effect may only be sustained for a few months. Another study showed that oil extracted from the borage plant had some properties similar to nonsteroidal anti-inflammatory drugs (NSAIDs), without gastrointestinal side effects. However, the best dosages and possible long-term side effects of these supplements have yet to be determined.

At this point, it is difficult to know the effect of supplements. There is also a phenomenon known as the *placebo effect.* In many research studies, some people are given the actual pill or treatment being tested, while others unknowingly receive a placebo, an inactive pill or treatment. Some people taking the placebo will experience the same results (reduced pain, for example) as the people taking the real drug, pointing to the potency of the power of suggestion.

For most types of supplements, unfortunately, solid scientific evidence is just not available. Few studies have been done to test supplements, and the studies that do exist usually don't stand up to rigorous scientific examination. In addition, these types of treatments are not regulated and tested in the same way that pharmaceutical products are to ensure that they are both safe and effective. Finally, there are few or no purity standards or quality control mechanisms in place.

It may seem like a paradox, but most pills that are labeled as "natural" contain chemicals that are processed, just like drugs. It's true that "natural" substances are chemicals found in the body normally, while drugs are chemicals that are not normally found in the body. But the chemicals in drugs are tested extensively for safety and purity, while the "natural" pills are not tested on the same level. It's not that you shouldn't consider "natural" remedies, but you should be aware of the concerns.

If you do decide to try an herbal extract, dietary supplement or other "natural" remedy, you should proceed with caution and keep the following points in mind:

• **Ask questions.** Don't be afraid to ask your doctor, pharmacist or other health professionals for their opinion or a recommendation.
• **Buy wisely.** When purchasing a supplement, buy from a large company, pharmacy or health-food chain. They may have more stringent quality controls than small companies to maintain their good reputation.
• **Read labels carefully.** Be aware that no supplement can lawfully claim to treat, cure, diagnose or prevent disease. Look for products with the U.S.P. notation, indicating that the manufacturer followed standards established by the United States Pharmacopoeia.
• **Try products one at a time.** If you try only one you can keep track of its effect (or lack of effect). If you notice any side effects, stop taking the supplement right away.

COMMON SUPPLEMENTS USED FOR RA

There are numerous herbs, supplements and similar treatments touted as being beneficial for people with rheumatoid arthritis. But do they really work or are they a waste of your hard-earned dollars? It's hard to say. In most cases, these treatments have not been thoroughly, scientifically tested to see if they are truly effective in the fight against RA symptoms. In other words, there is no solid evidence that they really work – or even, in some cases, that they might not do more harm than good. But they might be beneficial for some people.

We urge you to be cautious when trying natural treatments for RA like the ones listed below. Why? Herbs and supplements are considered the same as food by the U.S. government. They may be sold without approval by the Food and Drug Administration (FDA) and do not have to undergo the same rigorous testing and sanctioning processes that drugs do. So you, the consumer, must use your own good judgment. *Talk to your doctor before trying any herb or supplement*, as these products may interact with your current prescription or over-the-counter drugs. It's important to get your doctor's approval before trying any new treatment. Do not rely on the websites or literature of companies that manufacture these treatments, the websites or literature of retailers that sell these treatments, or on hearsay. That could be dangerous to your health.

For more information on herbs and supplements, consult the website of the National Center for Complementary and Alternative Medicine, www.nccam.nih.gov, part of the National Institutes of Health. Legitimate studies will be reported there. You can also find information about herbs and supplements used for arthritis on www.arthritis.org.

Black Currant Oil: Oil derived from the black currant fruit's seeds. Supposed to lessen RA joint pain, stiffness and swelling. Available in capsule form.

Borage Oil: Oil derived from the seeds of the borage plant. Supposed to lessen RA joint pain, stiffness and swelling. Available in capsule form.

Boron: Trace mineral found in many foods and multivitamins. Supposed to have anti-inflammatory effects and may improve joint and bone health. Available in many pill forms or in natural foods.

Boswellia: Gum resin from bark of the Oswellia tree. Supposed to have anti-inflammatory effects and fight arthritis symptoms. Available in capsule or pill form.

Cat's Claw: Dried root bark of a Peruvian vine. Supposed to have anti-inflammatory effects. Available in many forms, including capsule, tablet and tea bag infusion.

Cayenne: Also known as red pepper or capsaicin, cayenne is a hot pepper whose oil is often used in topical creams. May temporarily relieve pain in small areas. Do not use with other heat sources, such as heating pads, as it may cause burns. Not for internal use. Available in cream form.

Collagen: Protein found in human and animal cartilage – supplement forms derived from animal only. Supposed to relieve pain, swelling, inflammation and stiffness. Available in capsule, tablet or powder form.

Curcumin: Pulverized root from the turmeric plant (the powder supplement is

Before Trying an Alternative Therapy

• Many alternative therapies are not regulated.
Before you decide to try one of these therapies, find out as much about it as you can. A good source of information is the National Center for Complementary and Alternative Medicine (NCCAM), www.nccam.nih.gov. For a free packet of information, write to the NCCAM Clearinghouse, P.O. Box 8218, Silver Spring, MD 20807-8218.

• Once you have information on a particular therapy, discuss it with your doctor.
He or she will be able to answer important questions such as "How will this affect my treatment plan overall?" and "Could this cause any problems by interacting with my medications?"

• If you decide to proceed, do so with caution.
Seek out a qualified practitioner. For example, there are licensing requirements by state and/or national boards in biofeedback, acupuncture and massage therapy.

• Consider the cost.
Many alternative therapies are expensive, forcing you to weigh your options carefully. Therapies such as massage may or may not be covered by insurance policies when recommended by a physician, so read your policy closely.

• Use good judgment.
If the practitioner makes unrealistic claims (such as, "It will cure your arthritis.") or suggests that you should discontinue your conventional treatment, consider it a strong warning that something is not right.

Adapted from: *Kids Get Arthritis Too.* Atlanta: Arthritis Foundation. May/June 1999.

also called turmeric), commonly used in cooking. Supposed to relieve pain, inflammation and stiffness. Available in capsule or powder form.

Devil's Claw: Plant found in southern Africa. Supposed to relieve pain and inflammation, as well as to aid digestion. Available in capsule, powder or tea leaf form.

Evening Primrose Oil: Seeds of a wildflower indigenous to America, containing gamma-linoleic (see below) acid. Supposed

to lessen RA joint pain, stiffness and swelling. Available in capsule form.

Fish Oil: Oil derived from cold-water fish such as salmon, herring, tuna, mackerel and halibut, as well as the traditional treatment cod-liver oil. Supposed to fight inflammation and morning stiffness, and reduce fatigue. Available in capsule or pill form, or through adding cold-water fish to diet.

Flaxseed: Seed of flax plant. Supposed to lessen stiffness and joint pain, and to "lubricate" joints. Available in seed, ground flour or meal, capsule or oil form.

Ginger: Dried or fresh root of *zingiber officinale* plant, or common gingerroot. Supposed to reduce inflammation and lessen joint pain, as well as protecting the stomach from ulcers and the gastrointestinal side effects of NSAIDs. Available in powder, extract, tincture, spice and oil form.

GLA: Gamma-linoleic acid, an omega-6 fatty acid found in supplements like black currant oil, borage oil and evening primrose oil (see earlier listings). Supposed to have anti-inflammatory effects and to ease joint pain and stiffness. Available in capsule or oil form; must be taken orally.

MSM: Sulfur compound found in many fruits, vegetables and grains, as well as naturally occurring in animals and humans. Supposed have anti-inflammatory and analgesic effects. Available in tablet and powder form, and can be taken orally or used topically.

Selenium: Essential mineral found in many multivitamins. Supposed to fight joint tenderness and pain, as well as inflammation. Can be toxic in larger doses than the body needs. Available in tablet form and in many multivitamins.

Stinging Nettle: Leaves and roots of the *urtica dioica* plant. Supposed to have anti-inflammatory effects and to ease aches and pains. Available in tea, tincture, extract or leaf form; can be used externally as a poultice.

Thunder God Vine: Roots and leaves of a vine found mostly in Asia, *tripterygium wilfordii*. Supposed to have anti-inflammatory and analgesic effects, as well as treating disorders of the immune system. Available in extract form.

Turmeric: See *curcumin* p. 184.

Willow Bark: Derived from the bark of the white willow tree, containing salicin, an ingredient chemically similar to the active in ingredient in aspirin and many NSAIDs. Supposed to have anti-inflammatory and analgesic effects. Available in extract, tea or tincture form, as well as in some topical creams.

Zinc Sulfate: Mineral found in many multivitamins. Supposed to improve joint swelling, stiffness and overall well-being. Available in multivitamin compounds in liquid, capsule, softgel or tablet form, as well as in foods such as oysters, meat, eggs, tofu and black-eyed peas.

PRAYER AND SPIRITUALITY

Many people believe that prayer and spirituality can help us cope with suffering, offer comfort in times of illness and depression, and perhaps even help in healing. Public opinion polls have shown that prayer is one of the most commonly used alternative therapies for arthritis. Indeed, research in behavioral medicine suggests that the interactions of the mind, body and spirit can have powerful effects on our health. But very few published scientific studies have examined the effects of prayer and spirituality.

It may be difficult to measure the effects of prayer and faith on health. One way scientists have approached the issue is to study people who regularly attend religious services, compared with others who do not. Such studies suggest that people who attend religious services tend to live longer, take better care of their health and recover more quickly from illnesses and depression. However, skeptics contend that these studies really show the benefits of companionship and community, not religion.

People have found comfort, meaning and inspiration from prayer and other spiritual practices for thousands of years. Adding or deepening the spiritual aspects in your life could be good for you and arthritis, and – unless you abandon your medication and/or other components of your treatment program – certainly won't hurt you. Just remember that prayer alone will not "cure" your arthritis.

MISCELLANEOUS THERAPIES

Many other types of alternative and complementary therapies are available. In fact, it seems new ones are reported every week. They range from the probably harmless (copper bracelets) to the potentially harmful (bee sting therapy). For a more in-depth look at therapies targeted to people with arthritis, check out *The Arthritis Foundation Guide to Alternative Therapies*, published in 1999.

Talking to Your Doctor About Your Options

Doctors are more willing to discuss the use of alternative and complementary therapies with their patients than ever before, in part because they realize that their patients are using them, with or without a doctor's advice. Also, there is strong evidence that many complementary therapies can and do relieve some of the symptoms of arthritis, at least in the short-term.

If your doctor seems reluctant to talk about alternatives to traditional medical treatment with you, don't give up. Tell your doctor that it is important to you to discuss this topic. Be insistent (but not confrontational). The following list of questions might help you open the lines of communication:

• Is this a therapy that might help my condition?
• Have you read any studies about or had experience with this type of therapy?
• Is this therapy controversial? Why (or why not)?
• What are the hazards of the therapy?
• Will there be any interaction between this therapy and the medications or other treatments you have prescribed for me?
• Where can I get more information on the therapy?

Remember, it's in your best interest to keep your doctor informed about your treatment decisions. He or she can't give you the best professional advice without knowing all of the treatments you are using – whether they are over-the-counter drugs, herbal remedies or exercise programs.

Making Smart Choices

Keeping in mind all we've discussed in this chapter, it's up to you to be a smart consumer (see box, p. 185) when it comes to the use of alternative and complementary therapies. Be realistic when assessing the benefits and drawbacks of such therapies. Based on what we know now, certain alternative/complementary practices can help ease some arthritis symptoms, improve your outlook and work with conventional medicine to enhance the effects of your arthritis treatment plan. However, these therapies cannot replace proven medical treatments, nor can they cure chronic disease.

Chapter 18

Good Living:

Creating a Healthy Lifestyle

We have come a long way in this book, and we've covered quite a bit of information — including information to help you understand more about rheumatoid arthritis, the modern treatments available at this time, and practical suggestions that may help make living with rheumatoid arthritis easier. In fact, you may be feeling overwhelmed by the sheer volume of it all, and wondering how you can ever pull it all together into a plan that works for you.

In this chapter, we will try to help you do just that: Take the information that pertains to you and use it to create your own wellness lifestyle. A wellness lifestyle is one in which you are committed to nourishing your body and mind. It includes attitudes and behaviors that help you achieve the highest possible physical, mental and spiritual well-being. Creating a wellness lifestyle is a cornerstone of being a successful self-manager.

Setting Reasonable Goals

Obviously, there are many components to learning to live well with arthritis, or any other chronic disease. And, as we have stressed throughout this book, no two people are alike and no one experiences rheumatoid arthritis in exactly the same way. Take a few moments to look back over the Table of Contents of this book. Some chapters may not apply to you right now. For example, your active disease may be well controlled by medication, so the chapter on surgery may

be of less interest to you at this point. Or perhaps you're into exercise and have already worked out what kinds of exercises make you feel better and which ones to avoid.

Now, jot down a few areas you feel you need to change in your life to achieve a wellness lifestyle. The key word here is "few." How many times have you made sweeping New Year's resolutions, only to break them in a couple of weeks and end up feeling guilty and defeated? Changing old habits and creating new ones is hard work. Most experts advise setting reasonable goals that you can live with, rather than trying to change everything in your life at once. An example of a reasonable goal might be something like "I will walk three times a week for 20 minutes," rather than "I will begin training to run the New York marathon!"

You may want to make copies of the form below and use them to draw up weekly contracts with yourself. This will help you set reasonable goals by listing the specific steps you will take to achieve each goal.

Once you accomplish these goals, you can either raise the bar (for example, walking 40 minutes instead of 20), or if you've reached a level that you're happy with, you can turn your attention to other areas.

Nourishing Your Mind and Spirit

When you're setting goals, don't forget about those that will help you keep a healthy mental, as well as physical, outlook. Taking the time to nourish your mind and spirit can lead to unexpected health benefits

Contract Form

THIS WEEK I WILL: **WEEK OF:**_____

This week I will <u>walk</u> (what) <u>around the block</u> (how much) <u>before lunch</u> (when) <u>three times</u> (how many).

What

How Much

When

How Many Days

How Certain Are You   *(On a scale of 0 to 10 with 0 being totally unsure and 10 being totally confident)*

Signature:

like less physical pain, something researchers have found repeatedly to be true for people with chronic diseases.

We aren't always taught how to nourish ourselves emotionally or spiritually. Sometimes, people are taught to do the exact opposite – to ignore their emotions or feelings. However, there are many ways, both big and small, that we can enrich our minds and spirits. Consider the following points to help support a healthy mental outlook.

• **Optimism.** Having the view that things in general are pretty good can help you live longer and reduce chronic stress. Expect good things to happen, and work toward them. Stop worrying so much! Live one day at a time and use relaxation techniques and healthy self-talk to counter pessimistic thoughts.

• **Humor.** Laughter really is good medicine. Author Norman Cousins refers to laughing as "internal jogging." Anything that makes you smile brings relief to your mind and spirit. Some research has shown that humor may even improve your immune function.

• **Sense of purpose.** Do you believe you have worth and that there is a purpose for your life and experiences? People who

Personally Speaking — Stories from real people with rheumatoid arthritis

Smelling the Roses, Watching the Clouds – Appreciating Life
by Suzie Hershman, Matawan, NJ

"I wake up to a beautiful spring day. The sun is shining, a warm breeze is blowing, squirrels are playing tag. A rabbit nibbles clover while the blue jay in the pine tree outside my window scolds him. All these things, in addition to walking, I used to take for granted.

"A few years ago, I had 'routine' hip replacement surgery and almost ended up being unable to walk. Several surgeries and thousands of hours of physical therapy later, I'm walking! The time span and length of my walks are still limited; I will never be as strong or as stable was I was before. This can be depressing. When I lose patience and feel like giving up, I talk to a friend who reminds me how far I've come, and how much better I'm doing. Often, I write lists of things I can or cannot do. I compare the recent lists with the old lists. Looking at the improvements I've made, written down on paper, makes them seem more tangible.

"I stop and smell the roses that my husband planted along our driveway. I admire the splendid pinks, reds and oranges in the setting sun. I look out my window while typing, and watch the billowy, white clouds float across the sky. There are many other wonderful things in my world that help me get through the tough days, as well as the good ones."

believe in themselves and in the meaning of their lives are happier, more satisfied and serene. This belief in one's self is a choice that occurs regardless of life circumstances.

• **Sense of control.** Do you feel hopeless or frustrated by your arthritis or by other challenges in your life? Given the same situation, some people will feel helpless, and others feel a sense of control or of confidence that they can influence their own well-being. Goal setting, problem solving, self-monitoring, and communicating your needs and feelings to others are all ways to help you regain a sense of control.

• **Social support.** Is your life filled with satisfying relationships and love? Do you feel that others understand your arthritis and the demands it places on you? Getting the support you need can be hard work. You need to be a friend to have a friend. You need to be willing to listen to others and communicate your own needs in a clear, direct way.

Taking Care of the Basics

To truly live well with rheumatoid arthritis, you should take steps toward healthy living in general. Most of these basics have already been discussed in this book, but they're worth repeating because they are such an important part of feeling healthy and in charge of your life. So keep them in mind as you build your wellness lifestyle:

• **Eat a healthful diet.** Most people with rheumatoid arthritis don't need to follow any special diet. However, you should try to follow the guidelines for a healthy diet described in Chapter 17, in the box on the next page, or explained in the USDA's food pyramid.

• **Get enough sleep.** Many people are sleep deprived due to the demands of work, family and other obligations. We rise early and don't get to bed until late. Lack of sleep increases stress levels and may decrease your body's immune activity. Review the suggestions in Chapter 16 for getting a good night's sleep.

• **Manage stress in healthy ways.** We've talked about ways to reduce stress levels and tips for handling those stresses that can't be eliminated (see Chapter 13). Resist the temptation to handle stress in unhealthy ways – such as overeating, over-indulging in alcohol or taking drugs – that will only increase stress in the long run.

• **Balance exercise and rest.** Getting regular exercise should be an important part of your wellness lifestyle, but don't forget to balance periods of activity with periods of rest. Taking a 20-minute "breather" may feel like a waste of time, but it may just give you the energy you need to make it through the day.

A Final Word: Making Time for Yourself

Too many people fall into the trap of doing everything that others expect of them but failing to leave enough time for themselves. However, research has shown that your use of time and your overall balance of activities can affect your health and satisfaction with life. Try using the Time Target at the end of this chapter to help you think about how satisfied

Guidelines for a Healthy Diet

Eat a variety of foods.

Maintain a healthy weight.

Cut down on fat and cholesterol consumption.

Eat plenty of vegetables, fruits and grain products.

Use sugar and salt in moderation.

Drink plenty of water – most experts recommend eight glasses per day.

If you drink alcohol, do so in moderation.

you are with the amount of time you now spend on activities such as hobbies, time alone or with friends, or other activities that are "just for you."

Look for patterns in the Time Target. Is your life balanced so that most or all of the "bull's eye" (the center circle) is colored in? Or do you have a lot of parts of the other circles colored in? Look for colored areas in these outer circles:

• **"Need Less" circle.** If you have a lot of this circle colored in, you may have trouble setting priorities or saying no to others. Are you feeling overwhelmed? If so, go back and read the strategies for dealing with fatigue in Chapter 16, and for using more effective self-management techniques in Chapter 13.
• **"Need More" circle.** Is it hard for you to ask for what you need? Do you need more from people in relationships? You may need to practice better planning so that you can spend

more time on more enjoyable activities. Remember to set goals, contract, problem solve and plan to get where you want to be.
• **"Not Important."** If you have colored five or more of the activities as "not important," this may be a sign that you are feeling depressed. If you've lost interest in many activities that you used to enjoy, if you've isolated yourself from friends, or if you feel like hurting yourself, seek professional help. Go back and review the sections on coping with stress and coping with depression in Chapter 13 for additional help.

It is important to find those things in life that uplift and bring joy and happiness to your life. This will take time, patience and determination, but if you can learn to balance each of the hassles in your life with uplifting activities, rheumatoid arthritis can become just a part of your life, not your whole life.

Remember: Aim for the bull's eye.

Targeting Your Time

Instructions: Read the names for each of the 12 items listed in the wedges of the circle below. Think about how satisfied you are with the time you now spend on each item. Color in the part of the wedge for each item that best describes how it fits into your life. For example, if you are satisfied with time spent on something, color the center part of the wedge, in the "OK" section. Otherwise, indicate by coloring whether you "need less" or "need more" of it, or if it is "not important" in your life.

HOW CLOSE ARE YOU TO THE BULL'S-EYE?

GOOD LIVING RESOURCES

The Arthritis Foundation: Helping People with Arthritis and Chronic Joint Symptoms

The Arthritis Foundation offers information and support for the nearly 70 million Americans affected by any of the more than 100 forms of arthritis and related conditions or chronic joint symptoms. Arthritis Foundation chapters and branch offices nationwide help support research, professional and community education programs, services for people with arthritis, government advocacy and fundraising activities.

The mission of the Arthritis Foundation is to improve lives through leadership in the prevention, control and cure of arthritis and related diseases. Local offices provide information and support to help people with arthritis lead healthier, more fulfilling lives.

Through the Arthritis Foundation website (www.arthritis.org), its toll-free telephone call center (800-283-7800) or at chapter and branch offices nationwide (you can find yours by logging onto the website or by calling the toll-free national number), people with arthritis, their families and physicians can learn more about the following resources:

- **Publications.** Six times a year, the Arthritis Foundation publishes the award-winning magazine *Arthritis Today,* which offers health and lifestyle news and features for any person with arthritis or a related condition. *Arthritis Today* also publishes special inserts and issues, including the annual *Buyer's Guide,* which contains information on hundreds of companies that offer products and services to help people with arthritis or related diseases. The Arthritis Foundation also publishes an array of free, educational brochures on a wide variety of arthritis-related topics, from specific diseases, lifestyle challenges, current medications and more. Some information is available in easy-to-read format, as well as in Spanish. In addition, the Arthritis Foundation publishes a line of more than 25 informative, in-depth books on arthritis and related topics, and several exercise videos.

- **Physician referral.** Most Arthritis Foundation chapters can provide a list of doctors in their area who specialize in the evaluation and treatment of arthritis and arthritis-related diseases.

- **Exercise programs.** The Arthritis Foundation sponsors a number of exercise programs, both land- and water-based. These exercise programs are designed to accommodate people with arthritis, and take physical limitations into consideration. Arthritis Foundation chapters and branch offices can provide up-to-date lists of classes in every community. Many communities offer walking clubs and other group exercise opportunities. In addition, the Arthritis Foundation produces videotapes of these exercise programs for home use.

- **Classes and Courses.** The Arthritis Foundation offers formal group meetings to help people with various forms of arthritis gain the knowledge, skills and confidence they need to actively manage their conditions. Courses focus on proper exercises, medications, relaxation techniques, pain management, dealing with depression, nutrition, nontraditional treatments and doctor-patient relations.

- **Information Hotline and Website.** The Arthritis Foundation's toll-free information and resource line, 800/283-7800, and its website, www.arthritis.org, offer a wide variety of resources for people with arthritis and chronic joint symptoms. Information is also available in Spanish.

GLOSSARY

acupressure: Eastern medicine technique in which pressure is applied to specific sites along energy pathways called meridians.

acupuncture: Eastern medicine technique in which needles are used to puncture the body at specific sites along energy pathways called meridians.

acute illness: Disease that can be severe, but is of short duration, unlike chronic illness.

acute pain: See pain.

adrenal glands: Glands located near the kidneys. These glands secrete a variety of hormones, including glucocorticoids.

adrenaline: A hormone that increases the heart and respiration rate when we feel frightened, threatened or angry, preparing us to flee to safety, or stand and fight.

aerobic: An activity designed to increase oxygen consumption by the body, such as aerobic exercise or aerobic breathing.

alternative therapy: Any practice or substance outside the realm of conventional medicine.

American College of Rheumatology (ACR): An organization that provides a professional, educational, and research forum for rheumatologists across the country. Among its functions is helping determine what symptoms and signs define the various types of rheumatic disease diagnoses and what the appropriate treatments are for those diagnoses.

analgesic: Drugs used to help relieve pain.

anemia: A condition marked by a reduction in the number of red blood cells, amount of hemoglobin in the blood, or total blood volume.

anemia, iron deficiency: Anemia resulting from a greater demand on the stored iron than can be supplied.

anemia, pernicious: Anemia resulting from a lack of vitamin B12; it is associated with absence of hydrochloric acid in the stomach.

anesthesia: Chemicals that induce a partial or complete loss of sensation. Used to perform surgery and other medical procedures.

anesthesiologist: A physician specializing in the administration of anesthesia.

ankylosing spondylitis: Form of arthritis that primarily affects the joints and ligaments of the spine, marked by pain and stiffness. Can result in fusion of joints and bones, leading to rigidity.

antibody: A specialized protein that neutralizes *antigens,* or foreign substances, in the body.

antigen: A foreign substance that begins an immune reaction in the body.

antinuclear antibody test: Test used to detect presence of abnormal antibodies.

arthritis: From the Greek word "arth" meaning "joint," and the suffix "itis" meaning "inflammation." It generally means involvement of a joint from any cause, such as infection, trauma or inflammation.

arthrodesis: A surgical procedure involving the fusing of two bones.

arthroplasty: A surgical procedure to replace a joint with an artificial one.

arthroscopic surgery: A type of surgery using

an instrument, called an arthroscope, consisting of a thin tube with a light at one end, inserted into the body through a small incision, and connected to a closed-circuit television.

aspiration: The removal of a substance by suction. Technique used to remove fluid from an inflamed joint, both to relieve pressure and to examine the fluid.

autoantibody: antibodies acting against the body's own tissues.

autoimmune disorder: An illness in which the body's immune system mistakenly attacks and damages tissues of the body. There are many types of autoimmune disorders, including arthritis and the rheumatic diseases.

biologic response modifiers: Drugs that target the specific components of the immune system that contribute to disease. Includes etanercept and infliximab.

biomedical model: Traditional model of medical care, based on the principle of identifying a single cause and cure for each disease.

biopsychosocial model: More recent model of medical care, where patient's self-management plays a part in treatment of chronic disease, and where biological, psychological and socioeconomic factors are considered influential to the disease's outcome.

body mechanics: The structures and methods with which your body moves and performs physical tasks.

bone densitometry: Imaging study used to measure bone density, particularly in diagnosing osteoporosis.

bunion: Inflammation, enlargement and malalignment of the joint of the great toe.

bursa: A small sac located between a tendon and a bone. The bursae (plural for bursa) reduce friction and provide lubrication. See also bursitis.

bursitis: Inflammation of a bursa (see *bursa* above), which can occur when the joint has been overused or when the joint has become deformed by arthritis. Bursitis makes it painful to move or put pressure on the affected joint.

C-reactive protein: Protein that when found in elevated levels in the body is an indication of inflammation.

capsaicin: A chemical contained in some hot peppers. Capsaicin gives these peppers their "burn" and has painkilling properties. It is available in nonprescription creams that can be rubbed on the skin over a joint to relieve pain.

cartilage: A firm, smooth, rubbery substance that provides a gliding surface for joint motion, and prevents bone-on-bone contact.

chiropodist: a doctor with particular training in the care of the feet. Also called podiatrist.

chronic illness: Disease that is of a long duration, such as rheumatoid arthritis.

chronic pain: Pain that is constant or persists over a long period of time, perhaps throughout life. See pain.

circadian rhythm: The daily, monthly and seasonal schedules on which living things carry out essential biologic tasks, such as eating, digesting, eliminating, growing and resting. Disruption of these rhythms –

when you travel rapidly across time zones (promoting "jet lag"), for example – has a negative and sometimes profound impact on performance and mood.

complementary therapy: Any practice or substance used in conjunction with traditional treatment.

control group: A group of people used as a standard for comparison in scientific studies.

cool-down exercises: A series of physical activities that allow your heart and respiration rates to return to normal after being elevated by exercise.

corticosteroids: see glucocorticoids.

cortisone: A hormone produced by the cortex of the adrenal gland. Cortisone has potent anti-inflammatory effects but can also have side effects. See also glucocorticoids.

Cox-2 inhibitors: Drugs that inhibit inflammation without the gastrointestinal side effects of traditional NSAIDs. Includes celecoxib and rofecoxib.

cytokines: Chemicals involved in the inflammatory response.

cytotoxic drugs: Chemicals that destroy cells or prevent their multiplication.

deconditioning: Loss of muscle mass and strength because of inactivity. See also reconditioning.

deep breathing: Drawing air into the lungs, filling them as much as possible, and then exhaling slowly. Performing this type of breathing rhythmically for a few minutes increases the amount of oxygen refreshing your brain and produces relaxation and readiness for mental tasks.

depression: A state of mind characterized by gloominess, dejection or sadness.

depression, clinical: A recognized mental illness in which the feelings of depression are severe, prolonged and hamper your ability to function normally.

dermatomyositis: See polymyositis.

disease: Sickness. Some physicians use this term only for conditions in which a structural or functional change in tissues or organs has been identified.

disorder: An ailment; an abnormal health condition.

DMARDs: Disease modifying anti-rheumatic drugs, used to slow or stop the progression of inflammatory joint disease. Includes methotrexate.

dose-pack: A package of glucocorticoid drugs with a tapered daily dosage.

double-blind studies: A method used in scientific studies to compare one intervention (such as a new medication) with other interventions, or no intervention. In this method, the study participants and the persons evaluating the interventions are "blinded" — that is, they aren't told who is getting the intervention being tested — so their responses will not be influenced by their opinions or expectations of the intervention.

endorphins: Natural painkillers produced by the human nervous system that have qualities similar to opiate drugs. Endorphins are released during exercise and when we laugh.

endurance exercises: Exercises such as swimming, walking and cycling that use the large muscles of the body and are dependent on increasing the amount of oxygen that reaches the muscles. These exercises strengthen muscles and increase and maintain physical fitness.

enthesis: The place where the tendon inserts into the bone.

ergonomics: The study of human capabilities and limitations in relation to the work system, machine or task, as well as the study of the physical, psychological and social environment of the worker. Also known as "human engineering."

erosions: Small holes near the ends of bones.

erythrocyte sedimentation rate: A test measuring how fast red blood cells (erythrocytes) fall to the bottom of a test tube, indicating level of inflammation. Often called ESR or "sed rate."

fatigue: A general worn-down feeling of no energy. Fatigue can be caused by excessive physical, mental or emotional exertion, by lack of sleep, and by inflammation or disease.

Felty's syndrome: Form of rheumatoid arthritis marked by an enlargement of the spleen and a reduced number of white blood cells.

fibromyalgia: A noninfectious rheumatic condition affecting the body's soft tissue. Characterized by muscle pain, fatigue and nonrestorative sleep, fibromyalgia produces no abnormal X-ray or laboratory findings. It is often associated with headaches and irritable bowel syndrome.

flare: A term used to describe times when the disease or condition is at its worst.

flexibility exercises: Muscle stretches and other activities designed to maintain flexibility and to prevent stiffness or shortening of ligaments and tendons.

Food Labeling Act: Recent legal decree of the U.S. government mandating the type of information that must be given on food labels regarding nutritional content. This Act ensures that consumers will have easy-to-read fat, protein, fiber, carbohydrate and calorie content information, and more.

gate theory: A theory of how pain signals travel to the brain. According to this theory, pain signals must pass a "pain gate" that can be opened or closed by various positive (e.g., feelings of happiness) or negative (e.g., feelings of sadness) factors.

genetic predisposition: Susceptibility to a specific disease or illness caused by certain inherited characteristics.

glucocorticoids: A group of hormones including cortisol produced by the adrenal glands. They can also be synthetically produced (that is, made in a laboratory) and have powerful anti-inflammatory affects. These are sometimes called corticosteroids or steroids, but they are not the same as the dangerous performance-enhancing drugs that some athletes use to promote strength and endurance.

gout: Disease that occurs due to an excess of uric acid in the blood, causing crystals to deposit in the joint, leading to pain and inflammation.

grief: Feelings of loss; acute sorrow.

guided imagery: A method of managing pain

and stress. Following the voice of a "guide," an audiotape or videotape, or one's own internal voice, attention is focused on a series of images that lead one's mind away from the stressor or pain.

H2 blockers: Compounds that act by blocking receptors in the stomach that lead to the production of acid.

hammer toes: A specific type of joint malalignment of the toes seen in rheumatoid arthritis.

helplessness: The concept of not feeling in control of your life or your health.

hematocrit: The percentage of red blood cells found in blood.

hemoglobin: The protein in red blood cells that carries oxygen from the lungs to the tissues.

hormones: Concentrated chemical substances produced in the glands or organs that have specific – and usually multiple – regulatory effects to carry out in the body.

illness: Poor health; sickness.

immune response: Activation of the body's immune system.

immune system: Your body's complex biochemical system for defending itself against bacteria, viruses, wounds and other injuries. Among the many components of the system are a variety of cells (such as T cells), organs (such as the lymph glands) and chemicals (such as histamine and prostaglandins).

inflammation: A response to injury or infection that involves a sequence of biochemical reactions. Inflammation can be generalized, causing fatigue, fever, and pain or tenderness all over the body. It can also be localized, for example, in joints, where it causes swelling and pain. In rheumatoid arthritis, inflammation is not caused by injury or infection, but is part of an autoimmune reaction.

internist: A physician who specializes in internal medicine; sometimes called a primary-care physician.

isometric exercises: Exercises that build the muscles around joints by tightening the muscles without moving the joints.

isotonic exercises: Exercises that strengthen muscles by moving the joints.

joint: The place or part where one bone connects to another.

joint count: An examination done by a doctor to determine the number of joints that are affected by arthritis.

joint malalignment: When joints are not aligned properly, due to joint damage.

joint replacement surgery: Also known as arthroplasty, a surgical procedure involving the reconstruction or replacement (with a man-made component) of a joint.

ligament: Flexible band of fibrous tissue that connects bones to one another.

locus: The site of a gene on a chromosome.

lupus (systemic lupus erythematosus): The term used to describe an inflammatory connective tissue autoimmune disease that can involve the skin, joints, kidneys, blood and other organs, and is associated with antinuclear antibodies.

malalignment, joint: When joints are not aligned properly, due to joint damage.

massage: A technique of applying pressure, friction or vibration to the muscles, by hand or using a massage appliance, to stimulate circulation and produce relaxation and pain relief.

massage therapist: One who has completed a program of study and is licensed to perform massage.

meditation: A sustained period of deep inward thought, reflection and openness to inspiration.

meridians: Energy pathways used in Eastern medicine, but that have no Western medicine counterparts.

morbidity (rate): The frequency or proportion of people with a particular diagnosis or disability in a given population.

MRI: Magnetic Resonance Imaging test, a scan used as a diagnostic aid.

muscle: Tissue that moves organs or parts of the body.

myalgia: Pain of the muscles.

narcotic: A class of drug that reduces pain by blocking signals traveling from the central nervous system to the brain. While narcotics have the potential to be addictive and are abused by some people, they can be used safely for effective pain relief under skilled medical supervision.

NSAID (nonsteroidal anti-inflammatory drug): A type of drug that does not contain steroids but is used to relieve pain and reduce inflammation.

nurse: A person who has received education and training in health care, particularly patient care.

nurse practitioner: A registered nurse with advanced training and emphasis in primary care.

objective: Capable of being observed or measured; for example, infection can be objectively observed by the presence of bacteria in a blood test or culture test. See also subjective.

occupational therapist: A health professional who teaches patients to reduce strain on joints while doing everyday activities.

orthopaedic surgeon: A surgeon who specializes in diseases of the bone.

orthopaedist: A physician who specializes in diseases of the bone.

osteoarthritis: A disease causing cartilage breakdown in certain joints (spine, hands, hips, knees) resulting in pain and deformity.

osteoporosis: A disease that causes bones to lose their mass and break easily.

osteotomy: A surgical procedure involving the cutting of bone, usually performed in cases of severe joint malalignment.

pain: A sensation or perception of hurting, ranging from discomfort to agony, that occurs in response to injury, disease or functional disorder. Pain is your body's alarm system, signaling that something is wrong. *Acute* pain is temporary and related to nerve endings stimulated by tissue damage and improves with healing. *Chronic* pain may be mild to severe but persists due to prolonged tissue damage or due to pain impulses that keep the pain gate open.

palindromic rheumatism: Self-limited attacks of joint inflammation that occur every few weeks or months, then subside after a few days. About one half of people who experience palindromic rheumatism go on to develop chronic rheumatoid arthritis.

pediatrician: A physician with special training who specializes in the diagnosis, treatment and prevention of childhood and adolescent illness.

pediatric rheumatologist: See rheumatologist.

peptic ulcer: A benign (not cancerous) lesion in the stomach or duodenum that may cause pain, nausea, vomiting or bleeding. Such lesions can be caused by nonsteroidal anti-inflammatory drugs such as aspirin or ibuprofen.

pericarditis: Inflammation of the lining surrounding the heart.

pharmacist: A professional licensed to prepare and dispense drugs.

physiatrist: A physician who continues training after medical school and specializes in the field of physical medicine and rehabilitation.

physical therapist: A person who has professional training and is licensed in the practice of physical therapy.

physical therapy: Methods and techniques of rehabilitation to restore function and prevent disability following injury or disease. Methods may include applications of heat and cold, assistant devices, massage, and an individually tailored program of exercises.

physician: A person who has successfully completed medical school and is licensed to practice medicine.

physician, family: See physician, primary care.

physician, general practitioner: See physician, primary care.

physician, primary care: Physician to whom a family or individual goes initially when ill or for a periodic health check. This physician assumes medical coordination of care with other physicians for the patient with multiple health concerns.

physician's assistant: A person trained, certified and licensed to assist physicians by recording medical history and performing the physical examination, diagnosis and treatment of commonly encountered medical problems under the supervision of a licensed physician.

placebo effect: The phenomenon in which a person receiving an inactive drug or therapy experiences a reduction in symptoms.

platelets: Small cells that participate in the formation of blood clotting.

podagra: Gout occurring in the big toe.

podiatrist: A health professional who specializes in care of the foot. Formerly called a chiropodist.

polyarthritis: Arthritis affecting many joints.

polymyositis: Disease in which inflammation occurs primarily in the muscles, leading to muscle weakness and permanent muscle damage. Often associated with dermatomyositis, a condition marked by skin rashes.

Prosorba column: Treatment in which certain antibodies associated with rheumatoid arthritis are removed from the blood using a special filtering machine.

proton pump inhibitors: Drugs that block the secretion of acid into the stomach, used to protect the stomach against the gastrointestinal side effects associated with NSAIDs.

psoriatic arthritis: A condition in which psoriasis (a common skin disease) occurs in conjunction with the inflammation of arthritis.

psychiatrist: A physician who trains after medical school in the study, treatment and prevention of mental disorders. A psychiatrist may provide counseling and prescribe medicines and other therapies.

psychologist: A trained professional, usually a PhD rather than an MD, who specializes in the mind and mental processes, especially in relation to human and animal behavior. A psychologist may measure mental abilities and provide counseling.

psychosomatic: Pertaining to the link between the mind (psyche) and the body (soma).

pulmonary fibrosis: Scarring of the lungs, leading to shortness of breath.

radiograph: An X-ray.

range of motion (ROM): The distance and angles at which your joints can be moved, extended and rotated in various directions.

Raynaud's phenomenon: Restriction of blood flow to the fingers, toes, or (rarely) to the nose or ears, in response to cold or emotional upset. This results in temporary blanching or paleness of the skin, tingling, numbness and pain.

reconditioning: Restoring or improving muscle tone and strength with appropriate and balanced exercise, nutrition and rest. See also deconditioning.

rehabilitation counselor: A person who guides physical and mental rehabilitation.

relaxation: A state of release from mental or physical stress or tension.

remission: The term used to describe a period when symptoms of a disease or condition improve or even disappear.

remodeling: The regrowth of bone around an artificial joint.

resection: Surgical procedure involving removing all or part of a bone.

resection arthroplasty: A surgical procedure in which resection is done in conjunction with arthroplasty.

revision: A surgical procedure to replace an artificial joint.

rheumatic disease: A general term referring to conditions characterized by pain and stiffness of the joints or muscles. The American College of Rheumatology currently recognizes over 100 rheumatic diseases. The term is often used interchangeably with "arthritis" (meaning joint inflammation), but not all rheumatic diseases affect the joints or involve inflammation.

rheumatoid arthritis: A chronic, inflammatory autoimmune disease in which the body's protective immune system turns on the body and attacks the joints, causing pain, swelling and deformity.

rheumatoid factor: An abnormal antibody often found in blood of people with rheumatoid arthritis.

rheumatoid nodules: Lumps of tissue that form under the skin, often over bony areas exposed to pressure, such as on the fingers or around the elbow.

rheumatologist: A physician who pursues

additional training after medical school and specializes in the diagnosis, treatment and prevention of arthritis and other rheumatic disorders.

rheumatologist, pediatric: A rheumatologist who specializes in the diagnosis, treatment, and prevention of arthritis or other rheumatic diseases in children and adolescents.

salycilates: A subcategory of NSAIDs, including aspirin.

scleritis: Inflammation of the eyes.

scleroderma: A connective tissue disease characterized by a tightening of the skin, and a discoloration of the hands when exposed to cold (known as Raynaud's phenomenon). Can affect internal organs as well.

scleromalacia perforans: Permanent eye damage caused by severe inflammation

self-efficacy: The concept of a person having emotional control in reaction to events in their life, such as a chronic illness.

self-help: Any course, activity, or action that you do for yourself to improve your circumstances or ability to cope with a situation.

self-management: The concept of a person having control of his or her disease and its management.

self-talk: The voice in your head that you use to talk to yourself, out loud or in thought.

shared epitope: Genetic marker that approximately two-thirds of people with rheumatoid arthritis have.

Sjögren's syndrome: Syndrome affecting the salivary and lacrimal (tear-producing) glands, leading to dry eyes and dry mouth.

skeletal muscles: The voluntary muscles that are primarily involved in moving parts of the body. "Voluntary" in this sense refers to muscles that move in response to our decisions to walk, bend, grasp and so on, as opposed to muscles such as the heart, which do their work without our willful direction.

social worker: A person who has professional training and is licensed to assist people in need by helping them capitalize on their own resources and connecting them with social services (for example, home nursing care or vocational rehabilitation).

soft-tissue rheumatism: Pertaining to the many rheumatic conditions affecting the soft (as opposed to the hard or bony) tissues of the body. Fibromyalgia is one type of soft-tissue rheumatism. Others are bursitis, tendinitis and focal myofascial pain.

spontaneous remission: A somewhat rare disappearance of symptoms of rheumatoid arthritis, usually occurring in the early stage of disease.

steroids: A group name for lipids (fat substances) produced in the body and sharing a particular type of chemical structure. Among these are bile acids, cholesterol, and some hormones. Not the same as anabolic steroids, drugs synthesized from testosterone (the male sex hormone), and used by some athletes to promote strength and endurance.

strain: Injury to a muscle, tendon or ligament by repetitive use, trauma or excessive stretching.

strengthening exercises: Exercises that help maintain or increase muscle strength. See also isometric exercises and isotonic exercises.

stress: The body's physical, mental and chemical reactions to frightening, exciting, dangerous or irritating circumstances.

stressor: Factors that cause stress in your life.

symmetric arthritis: Arthritis affecting the same joints on both sides of the body.

syndrome: A collection of symptoms and/or physical findings that characterize a particular abnormal condition or illness.

synovectomy: Surgical removal of the synovium, or the lining of the joint.

synovitis: Inflammation of the lining of the joint.

synovium: The lining of the joint.

synovial fluid: The fluid found in the joint.

systemic disease: A disease that may affect more than one system in the body.

target heart rate: The number of heartbeats per minute that people want to reach during exercise in order to gain maximum benefits. Because the normal heart rate changes as we age, target heart rates are grouped by age.

tendinitis: Inflammation of a tendon.

tendon: A cord of dense, fibrous tissue uniting a muscle to a bone.

TENS: a treatment for pain involving a small device that directs mild electric pulses to nerves in the painful area.

teratogenic: Causing the malformation of a fetus.

thrombocytopenia: Decreased number of platelets.

tissue: A collection of similar cells that act together to perform a specific function in the body. The primary tissues are epithelial (skin), connective (ligaments and tendons), bone, muscle and nervous.

titer: A standard of strength per volume or units per volume.

trochanteric bursitis: Irritation of the trochanteric bursa, which is located on the bony prominence of the femur or thigh. See also bursitis.

Type I disease: Term used in rheumatoid arthritis to describe a case where a person meets certain criteria or shows symptoms of the disease for a short period of time, but these symptoms do not last long or progress in severity.

Type II disease: Term used in rheumatoid arthritis to describe a case where a person meets the criteria for the disease, experiences inflammation in symmetrical joints for longer than six months, and does not experience spontaneous remission of symptoms. A mild disease course that can be controlled with less aggressive therapy.

Type III disease: Most severe form of rheumatoid arthritis, with greater severity of symptoms than Type II disease, requiring aggressive therapy.

uric acid: Substance formed when the body breaks down waste products called *purines.* Uric acid crystals deposited in the joints cause gout.

urinalysis: Test done on the urine to detect levels of sugar, protein or abnormal cells.

vasculitis: Inflammation of the blood vessels.

visual analogue scale: A tool used to measure subjective feelings such as pain on a scale of 0 to 10 or 0 to 100.

visualization: A method of thinking that engages the imagination to help you achieve a goal.

warm-up: Gentle movement to warm up the muscles before performing stretches and more strenuous exercise.

INDEX

INDEX

INDEX

INDEX

INDEX

INDEX

ow You Have Two Great Ways to Get the ward-Winning Magazine, *Arthritis Today*!

1 Subscribe Today and Save 46% Off the Cover Price!

Subscribe and receive *Arthritis Today*, which is chock-full of the latest and most reliable advice you can get from the experts you trust at the Arthritis Foundation. In each information-packed issue you'll find:

• Top strategies for lowering the cost of medications
• Up-to-date information on arthritis drugs, therapies and nutritional supplements
• Ways to feel better, eat better and live better every day.

Just call 1-800-283-7800 to receive a year's subscription (6 issues) for just $12.95 and mention this code (A410GL).

OR

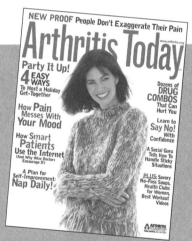

2 Get MORE for Your Money – Become a Member!

Become a member of the Arthritis Foundation and keep up with the latest news and research! As a member you will receive...

1 year's (6 issues) subscription to *Arthritis Today*
Arthritis Today Drug Guide, packed with information on hundreds of medications, ir side effects and more
sonalized membership card
mbers-only 10% discount on all books and videos
ecial announcements about self-help & education programs
cess to the Arthritis Specialists Referral List
ecial updates on cutting-edge arthritis research

Just call 1-800-283-7800 and become a member of the Arthritis Foundation for a minimum donation of $20.00 and mention this code (42393P20).

NEW! Do You Need Surgery?

ALL YOU NEED TO KNOW ABOUT
JointSurgery
By Mary Anne Dunkin

Preparing for Surgery,
Recovery and an
Active New Lifestyle

Important Items to Discuss With Your Doctor

AN OFFICIAL PUBLICATION OF THE ARTHRITIS FOUNDATION

All This FOR ONLY $19.95

You've probably tried a variety of drugs, creams, heating pads and exercises, but the pain just won't go away... and it only gets harder to do the things you love to do. You're asking yourself...

"Is it time for joint replacement surgery?"

Now more than ever, people with painful, debilitating arthritis are having joint replacements and other types of joint surgery on their knees, hips, shoulders and more. If you are one of the thousands of Americans each year who consider surgery, get the facts now with this brand-new book from the Arthritis Foundation!

With ***All You Need To Know About Joint Surgery: Get Ready for Surgery, Recovery and an Active New Lifestyle*** you will:
Discover the newest surgical techniques used by doctors to fight pain
See what really happens in the operating room
Learn easy steps you can take to make surgery more successful
Know when it's OK to delay surgery
Get tips for a successful recovery so you can get back into life!

Get the facts on:

- What type of surgery you need
- Risk factors you should know
- New techniques for replacing joints
- Keys to a smoother recovery

Are you ready for surgery? Get ready! Order ***All You Need To Know About Joint Surgery*** Now!

TO ORDER CALL 1-800-207-8633
(M-F 8 A.M. – 5 P.M. EST)
OR VISIT www.arthritis.org

ARTHRITIS FOUNDATION®
Take Control. We Can Help.™

Promotional code:BKRA04

What's Wrong With My Back?

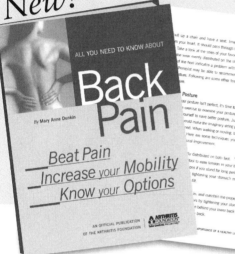

New!

ALL YOU NEED TO KNOW ABOUT

Back Pain

By Mary Anne Dunkin

Beat Pain
Increase *your* Mobility
Know *your* Options

AN OFFICIAL PUBLICATION
OF THE ARTHRITIS FOUNDATION

All This FOR ONLY $19.95

It's sore, tight. You can't sleep or find relief. After a few days, the pain gets worse…so bad that you have to miss a day of work. **What's wrong?**

You're experiencing **BACK PAIN**, one of the most common health problems in America today. For people of all ages, back pain is serious pain – and it requires serious attention from you and your doctor.

But what can you do about your back pain?

Now more than ever, there's a great deal you and your doctor can do to fight your back pain. Get all the latest treatments, techniques and prevention tips in a brand-new book from the Arthritis Foundation, *All You Need To Know About Back Pain: Beat Pain, Increase Your Mobility, Know Your Options.*

Are you ready to tell back pain to "back off"?
Order *All You Need To Know About Back Pain* today and find out how!

Get the facts on:

- The latest powerful drugs for your back

- Easy lifestyle changes to help you prevent back problems

- The truth about back surgery

- Alternative therapies that may really work for you

- New techniques to conquer your pain without pills